HIV/AIDS – Medical, Social and Psychological Aspects

HIV/AIDS

Pathophysiology, Prevention and Treatment

HIV/AIDS – MEDICAL, SOCIAL AND PSYCHOLOGICAL ASPECTS

Additional books and e-books in this series can be found on Nova's website under the Series tab.

HIV/AIDS – MEDICAL, SOCIAL AND PSYCHOLOGICAL ASPECTS

HIV/AIDS

PATHOPHYSIOLOGY, PREVENTION AND TREATMENT

ETHEL K. HEBERT
EDITOR

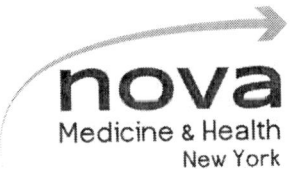

Copyright © 2020 by Nova Science Publishers, Inc.

All rights reserved. No part of this book may be reproduced, stored in a retrieval system or transmitted in any form or by any means: electronic, electrostatic, magnetic, tape, mechanical photocopying, recording or otherwise without the written permission of the Publisher.

We have partnered with Copyright Clearance Center to make it easy for you to obtain permissions to reuse content from this publication. Simply navigate to this publication's page on Nova's website and locate the "Get Permission" button below the title description. This button is linked directly to the title's permission page on copyright.com. Alternatively, you can visit copyright.com and search by title, ISBN, or ISSN.

For further questions about using the service on copyright.com, please contact:
Copyright Clearance Center
Phone: +1-(978) 750-8400   Fax: +1-(978) 750-4470   E-mail: info@copyright.com

NOTICE TO THE READER

The Publisher has taken reasonable care in the preparation of this book, but makes no expressed or implied warranty of any kind and assumes no responsibility for any errors or omissions. No liability is assumed for incidental or consequential damages in connection with or arising out of information contained in this book. The Publisher shall not be liable for any special, consequential, or exemplary damages resulting, in whole or in part, from the readers' use of, or reliance upon, this material. Any parts of this book based on government reports are so indicated and copyright is claimed for those parts to the extent applicable to compilations of such works.

Independent verification should be sought for any data, advice or recommendations contained in this book. In addition, no responsibility is assumed by the Publisher for any injury and/or damage to persons or property arising from any methods, products, instructions, ideas or otherwise contained in this publication.

This publication is designed to provide accurate and authoritative information with regard to the subject matter covered herein. It is sold with the clear understanding that the Publisher is not engaged in rendering legal or any other professional services. If legal or any other expert assistance is required, the services of a competent person should be sought. FROM A DECLARATION OF PARTICIPANTS JOINTLY ADOPTED BY A COMMITTEE OF THE AMERICAN BAR ASSOCIATION AND A COMMITTEE OF PUBLISHERS.

Additional color graphics may be available in the e-book version of this book.

Library of Congress Cataloging-in-Publication Data

Names: Hebert, Ethel K., editor.
Title: HIV/AIDS: pathophysiology, prevention and treatment / Ethel K. Hebert, editor.
Identifiers: LCCN 2020019487 (print) | LCCN 2020019488 (ebook) | ISBN 9781536179231 (paperback) | ISBN 9781536179927 (adobe pdf)
Subjects: LCSH: AIDS (Disease)--Pathophysiology. | HIV infections--Pathophysiology. | AIDS (disease)--Treatment. | HIV infections--Treatment.
Classification: LCC RC606.6 .H55 2020 (print) | LCC RC606.6 (ebook) | DDC 616.97/92--dc23
LC record available at https://lccn.loc.gov/2020019487
LC ebook record available at https://lccn.loc.gov/2020019488

Published by Nova Science Publishers, Inc. † *New York*

Contents

Preface		vii
Chapter 1	Depression and Anxiety in People Living with HIV/AIDS: Prevalence, Impact and Management *Suprakash Chaudhury, Ajay K Bakhla, Rajiv Saini, Mahesh Thakur and Daniel Saldanha*	1
Chapter 2	Socio-Psychological Determinants of Dental Care for Patients With HIV *Anastasiya Sergeevna Belyakova, Marina Vladlenovna Kozlova, Igor Vladimirovich Pchelin and Kirill Aleksandrovich Barsky*	69
Chapter 3	Management of Hepatitis C Virus in Patients Coinfected with HIV *Soha Freidy and Olga M. Klibanov*	81
Chapter 4	Prevention of HIV/AIDS among Youth *Todd Mamutle Maja*	97
Chapter 5	HIV Treatment as Prevention *Zanesha Jeter and Olga M. Klibanov*	137
Index		155

Preface

HIV/AIDS: Pathophysiology, Prevention and Treatment first discusses how depression and anxiety occur more frequently in people living with HIV/AIDS than in the general population. Anxiety and depression increase the morbidity of HIV by causing poor adherence to treatment, increased risk for suicide, greater chance for recurrence and various other significant mechanisms.

The authors present an analysis of sociological research showing the prevalence of stigma and discrimination against patients with HIV infection at the dental office. Fear of stigma is a key factor in reducing the willingness to disclose HIV status.

The recommended treatment for chronic hepatitis C virus infection with HIV coinfection is reviewed, focusing on the pharmacokinetics and pharmacology of drug-drug interactions between antiretroviral therapy and direct-acting antivirals.

Insight on the long road towards the eradication of HIV/AIDS is discussed in an effort to achieve sustainable development goals and targets by 2030. Studies conducted in relation to biomedical, structural, behavioural and technological interventions are cited to substantiate this discussions.

The closing chapter outlines updated recommendations guiding healthcare professionals to employ treatment as prevention. A discussion of the public health measures necessary to promote the success of treatment as prevention is also included.

Chapter 1 - An online literature search was carried out for articles related to HIV, depression, anxiety, prevalence, impact and treatment and about 200 articles were reviewed. It was found that depression and anxiety occur more frequently in people living with HIV/AIDS (PLWHA) than in the general population. The prevalence of depression and anxiety in PLWHA varies from 5.8% to 87% and 3% to 82.3%, respectively. The coexistence of these disorders has a major impact on PLWHA. Anxiety and depression increase the morbidity of HIV by poor adherence to treatment, increased risk for suicide, greater chance for recurrence and various other significant mechanisms. Studies indicate that effective management of anxiety and depression in PLWHA results in improved antiretroviral adherence, improved quality of life and increased survival. The management of anxiety and depression in PLWHA involves both pharmacological and nonpharmacological therapies. Benzodiazepines are only indicated for short periods of time. Clonazepam and lorazepam may be preferred due to lack of active metabolites and less drug–drug interactions. Selective serotonin reuptake inhibitors (SSRIs) are the preferred medication for long treatment of depression and anxiety. Though the different SSRIs are equally effective, sertraline, citalopram, and escitalopram are preferred in PLWHA to avoid interactions with antiretrovirals. Various psychotherapeutic interventions, including supportive psychotherapy, cognitive behavior therapy, interpersonal therapy, cognitive–behavioral-oriented group psychotherapy, experiential group psychotherapy, cognitive–behavioral stress management, stress management interventions, cognitive remediation, mindfulness-based therapy, and aerobic and resistance exercise have all been found to be useful in treating depression and anxiety in PLWHA. However, the comparative efficacy of the different nonpharmacological intervention for the management of anxiety and depression in PLWHA is yet to be determined.

Chapter 2 - The article presents an analysis of the data of sociological research, the purpose of which was to show the prevalence of stigma and discrimination against patients with HIV infection at the dental attendance. According to the results of a voluntary face-to-face individual anonymous survey of 1268 people, living with HIV, aged 18 years and older, there was a high level (66.7%) of stigma and discrimination in medical organizations providing dental care. Fear of stigma has been a key factor in reducing the willingness to disclose HIV status. 36.5% of respondents do not believe in the principle of confidentiality, they are out of concern for the disclosure of the diagnosis and the consequences associated with it. In this regard, only 22.4% of those interviewed for dental care reported having HIV infection. 29.9% of respondents were asked to take an HIV test - 60% of them voluntarily, 15% in an ultimatum form, 25% of patients were under pressure. A large number of acts of discrimination were revealed in the form of a negative attitude of a physician to patients with HIV infection (25% of cases) and refusal to treat oral diseases (41.7% of cases). According to the results of the survey, the doctors, having learned about the positive HIV status of the patient, refused mainly (94%) dental surgery (tooth extraction and dental implantation). There was a high proportion of people (64.2%) who postponed the visit to the dentist due to social concerns related to their HIV status. The data of the presented study actualize the necessity for development and realization of programs to eradicate stigma and discrimination towards people living with HIV in order to timely provide qualified medical dental care, improve oral health and the quality of life of these patients.

Chapter 3 - Hepatitis C virus (HCV) is a bloodborne disease transmitted via direct contact with HCV infected blood. Human immunodeficiency virus (HIV) can be transmitted through direct contact with HIV infected blood. Due to their common route of transmission, HCV infection is prevalent among HIV patients. About 62-80% of HIV patients are coinfected with HCV according to the Center for Disease Control and Prevention (CDC). The efficacy and safety profile of modern HCV therapy [i.e., direct-acting antivirals (DAA)] is similar among coinfected patients and mono-infected patients. However, HCV/HIV coinfected patients require continuous monitoring due to drug-drug interaction with DAAs and antiretroviral drugs. Treating HCV infection while maintaining adequate

HIV suppression could be challenging. For this reason, the American Association for the Study of Liver Diseases (AASLD) and the Infectious Disease Society of America (IDSA) published recommendations for managing and treating coinfected patients. This chapter will review the recommended treatment for chronic HCV infection with HIV coinfection, focusing on the pharmacokinetics and pharmacology of drug-drug interactions between antiretroviral therapy and DAAs.

Chapter 4 - Young people become sexually active at an early age and succumb to self-destructive behaviours such as alcohol and drug abuse, multiple sexual partners and unprotected sex resulting in unintentional pregnancies and sexually transmitted infections including HIV/AIDS.

Over 30% of all new HIV infections globally are estimated to occur among youth aged 15-24 years. In addition, children infected at birth grow into adolescents who have to deal with their HIV positive status, totalling 5 million youth living with HIV/AIDS. The greatest burden of HIV among young people is in the sub-Saharan Africa (SSA) (UNAIDS: 2016; WHO 2014, 2015).

Almost half of the 15-19 year olds who are living with HIV in the world, live in six countries, namely South Africa, Nigeria, Kenya, India, Mozambique and Tanzania. While HIV incidence and HIV- related deaths have decreased in other populations, in SSA, HIV-related deaths among youth continue to rise. Focusing on young people is likely to be the most effective approach to confronting the epidemic, particularly in high prevalence countries.

This chapter highlights HIV preventative measures which entail biomedical, behavioural and structural interventions as well as innovative technological strategies supported by literature sources from previous studies to provide evidence-based arguments.

In: HIV/AIDS
Editor: Ethel K. Hebert

ISBN: 978-1-53617-923-1
© 2020 Nova Science Publishers, Inc.

Chapter 1

DEPRESSION AND ANXIETY IN PEOPLE LIVING WITH HIV/AIDS: PREVALENCE, IMPACT AND MANAGEMENT

Suprakash Chaudhury[1,*], Ajay K. Bakhla[2], Rajiv Saini[3], Mahesh Thakur[4] and Daniel Saldanha[1]
[1]Department of Psychiatry, Dr. D. Y. Patil Medical College,
Dr. D. Y. Patil University, Pune, Maharshtra, India
[2]Department of Psychiatry, Rajendra Institute of Medical Sciences,
Ranchi, Jharkhand, India
[3]Department of Psychiatry, Command Hospital (EC),
Kolkata, West Bengal, India
[4]Department of Social Work, Karve Institute of Social Service,
Pune, Maharshtra, India

ABSTRACT

An online literature search was carried out for articles related to HIV, depression, anxiety, prevalence, impact and treatment and about 200

---

* Corresponding Author's Email: suprakashch@gmail.com.

articles were reviewed. It was found that depression and anxiety occur more frequently in people living with HIV/AIDS (PLWHA) than in the general population. The prevalence of depression and anxiety in PLWHA varies from 5.8% to 87% and 3% to 82.3%, respectively. The coexistence of these disorders has a major impact on PLWHA. Anxiety and depression increase the morbidity of HIV by poor adherence to treatment, increased risk for suicide, greater chance for recurrence and various other significant mechanisms. Studies indicate that effective management of anxiety and depression in PLWHA results in improved antiretroviral adherence, improved quality of life and increased survival. The management of anxiety and depression in PLWHA involves both pharmacological and nonpharmacological therapies. Benzodiazepines are only indicated for short periods of time. Clonazepam and lorazepam may be preferred due to lack of active metabolites and less drug–drug interactions. Selective serotonin reuptake inhibitors (SSRIs) are the preferred medication for long treatment of depression and anxiety. Though the different SSRIs are equally effective, sertraline, citalopram, and escitalopram are preferred in PLWHA to avoid interactions with antiretrovirals. Various psychotherapeutic interventions, including supportive psychotherapy, cognitive behavior therapy, interpersonal therapy, cognitive–behavioral-oriented group psychotherapy, experiential group psychotherapy, cognitive–behavioral stress management, stress management interventions, cognitive remediation, mindfulness-based therapy, and aerobic and resistance exercise have all been found to be useful in treating depression and anxiety in PLWHA. However, the comparative efficacy of the different nonpharmacological intervention for the management of anxiety and depression in PLWHA is yet to be determined.

Keywords: selective serotonin reuptake inhibitors, tricyclic antidepressants, benzodiazepines, cognitive behavior therapy, interpersonal therapy, mindfulness based therapy

INTRODUCTION

Acquired immune deficiency syndrome (AIDS) was initially identified in the USA in 1981 in young men who were homosexual and immunocompromised. The human immunodeficiency virus (HIV) was first detected in humans in 1983. Since then an estimated 74.9 million people have been infected with HIV and 32 million people died from AIDS-related illnesses all over the world (end 2018). An estimated 37.9 million people globally were living with HIV (end 2018). However, experts claim that the growth of the epidemic has stabilized. In the human body HIV is present in cell-free plasma, semen, cervical secretions, lymphocytes, cerebrospinal fluid, tears, saliva, urine and breastmilk. All these fluids may not transmit infection, as there are considerable variations in the concentration of virus in them. Semen, blood and cervical secretions are particularly infectious. Infection may follow exposure of mucosa to infected blood or body fluids. Transmission also occurs through the sharing of contaminated needles by injecting drug users, needle stick injuries, from mother to child in utero, at birth and through breastfeeding, transfusion of infected blood or organ transplantation. However, globally the commonest mode of transmission of HIV is through sexual intercourse (unprotected anal or vaginal). After entering the human body the HIV infects and kills the cells of the immune system, as a result of which the individual becomes more susceptible to various infections and malignancies. According to the World Health Organization (WHO) the infection can advance to a final stage of the acquired immunodeficiency syndrome (AIDS) in 10–15 years (Antiretroviral therapy can slow down the process even further). The diagnosis of HIV infection in people ≥18 months is defined by WHO as: "positive HIV antibody testing, which is confirmed by a second HIV antibody test relying on different antigens or of different operating characteristics; and/or positive virological test for HIV or its components confirmed by a second virological test obtained from a separate determination." [1, 2] Following the confirmation of a person's HIV-positive status, he or she has to make some life-changing decisions. Firstly, whether they should inform their significant other of their HIV-positive status. Secondly, about starting treatment and continuing it regularly. Finally, and most importantly about future sexual relations and whether they should have children. As a consequence of their decision, they may become isolated with reduced social support, may refuse treatment, or even develop psychiatric conditions such as anxiety and depression [3].

Four decades after its identification and especially with the widespread availability of combination ART being accessed by 24.5 million people globally (end June 2019), the status of HIV infection has greatly altered from a quick death sentence to a chronic condition. This has resulted in fewer deaths from AIDS and an increase in the number of people living with HIV/AIDS (PLWHA). Consequently there is greater awareness and concern about the psychological consequences of living with HIV infection. Psychological disturbances in PLWHA may vary from mild distress to major psychiatric disorders. Reports indicate that at all stages of HIV disease the prevalence of depression, anxiety, suicidal ideation and post-traumatic stress disorder are elevated. Depression is the commonest psychiatric disorder in PLWHA [4]. The prevalence of an anxiety disorder in PLWHA is also more common than in the general population [5]. Depression and anxiety adversely affect the adherence to ART, quality of life (QoL), and health-related QoL in PLWHA. In addition depression and anxiety are associated with increased morbidity and mortality in PLWHA [6-8]. On the other hand adequate treatment of depression and anxiety results in improvement in adherence to ART and overall functioning of PLWHA [9, 10].

HIV Related Mental Distress

Premorbid psychological and social adjustment, household income, culture, religion and family circumstances influence and can alter an individual's reaction to a diagnosis of HIV and subsequent adaptation to living with the diagnosis. These factors may contribute to HIV related mental distress. In addition, in their study, Chipimo and Fylkesnes [11] showed that HIV infection has both a direct and indirect effects on genesis of mental distress. HIV infection can cause direct organic brain tissue damage leading to the development of virtually any mental disorder, most commonly depression, anxiety, personality disorders and dementia. While the mechanisms explaining the development of these psychiatric disorders are not known, the presence of HIV-1 binding sites in the brain (chemokine receptors) allows HIV-1 to infect macrophages and microglia. Although neurons are not infected, they are injured by release of macrophage, microglial and astrocyte toxins along with viral proteins. These toxins produce overstimulation of the neurons, causing the creation of free radicals and excitotoxicity, and resultant death by apoptosis [12].

In a population having low awareness of own HIV sero-status and high prevalence of HIV infection, Chipimo and Fylkesnes [11] utilized a structural equation modeling (SEM) to establish the relationship between HIV infection and mental distress using maximum likelihood ratio as the method of estimation. The model indicated that underlying factors such as residence (rural or urban), level of education, marital status and age were inter-correlated as determinants for mental distress. Further, mental distress was found to be directly related to self-perceived risk and worry about being HIV infected, HIV sero-status and self-rated health [12].

There exists a complex relationship between HIV infection and depression. Undoubtedly depression is a consequence of HIV infection but it is also a risk factor [13, 14]. Factors contributing to depression in PLWHA include coping with the prospects of illness and death, neurobiological changes related to persistent central nervous system (CNS) infections due to HIV, comorbid disorders, social stigma, sexual dysfunction, and side effects of ART [15, 16]. In PLWHA depression often remains unrecognized and therefore untreated [17]. According to a meta-analytic study, the development of depression in PLWHA is neither associated with the sexual orientation of patients nor the stage of HIV infection [18].

The present work aims to summarize the recent research literature related to the prevalence, impact, and management of depression and anxiety in PLWHA. The literature review revealed that depression in PLWHA has been studied more often than anxiety. This bias is reflected in this review.

METHODS

Literature was searched online for articles related to HIV, depression, anxiety prevalence, impact and treatment during January and February 2020. A PubMed search was performed using the following paired phrases: "HIV Depression Anxiety," "HIV Depression Anxiety Prevalence," "HIV Depression Anxiety Impact," and "HIV Depression Anxiety Treatment," which returned 636, 232 and 790 articles respectively. In addition a Google search was carried out with the search term "HIV Depression Anxiety, Prevalence, Impact and Treatment." Abstracts of all the shortlisted articles were read to screen them. The full text of the selected articles were downloaded and reviewed. We preferred recently published articles over older ones. Many cross-references were also checked and the articles downloaded. Finally articles of the past ten years were tabulated. Articles were excluded if they were not written in English; full articles were not available or were of unrelated findings. Official documents from the WHO were also screened; in addition, some other articles were identified through Google and from the personal knowledge of the authors. In total, the findings of ~200 articles were reviewed.

RESULTS

Prevalence of Depression and Anxiety

For the present review we scrutinized ~60 and ~35 studies respectively, estimating the prevalence of depression and anxiety. As summarized in Table 1 and Table 2 there was a wide range of differences on the prevalence of depression and anxiety respectively across these studies. This was due to the use of different assessment methodologies and different definitions of anxiety and depression; using different diagnostic criteria like International Classification of Diseases or Diagnostic and Statistical Manual of Mental Disorders and their versions; use of different structured clinical interviews; and use of rating scales varying from self-report scales to clinician administered rating scales. The studies also vary in age range (only children and adolescents to adults), gender (only males, both gender, pregnant women, men who have sex with men, female sex workers) and stage of illness (asymptomatic to those with low CD4 counts). Studies also varied in their time duration about presence of symptoms: whether cross-sectional, past two weeks, past month, past year, or lifetime. This is important as the prevalence of psychiatric disorders is expected to increase as the time duration is extended [19].

The review found that the prevalence of depression in PLWHA is significantly higher than in the general population [19, 20]. A 2001 meta-analysis of ten studies stated that in PWLHA the prevalence of depression was ~10% as compared to only 5% in the general population; this was independent of sexual orientation of the individual and stage of illness [18]. Despite the high prevalence of depression in PLWHA, substantial percentage of patients with depression escape detection, and steps should be takes to improve identification.

The present review found wide variations in the prevalence of depression and anxiety among PWLHA across studies in the past decade. The prevalence rate of depression in HIV patients in different studies varied from 5.8% to 87% (Table 1). The 70 studies assessing depression were from all across the globe; sample sizes varied from 47 to 3816, used different methodologies, and different depression rating scales or questionnaires. The frequently used scales for assessment of depression were Hospital Anxiety and Depression Scale (13 studies), Patient Health Questionnaire 9 (11 studies), Beck Depression Inventory (8 studies) and Center for Epidemiologic Studies Depression Scale (7 studies).

Anxiety in PLWHA has generated less research interest, though clinical experience tells us that during the treatment of PLWHA comorbid anxiety is often missed and not treated. However the prevalence of anxiety in PLWHA is higher than in the general population. The prevalence rate of anxiety in HIV patients in different studies varied from 3% to 82.3% (Table 2). The 50 studies assessing anxiety were from all across the globe; sample sizes varied from 47 to 7834, used different methodologies, and different anxiety rating scales or questionnaires. The commonly used scales for the assessment of anxiety included Hospital Anxiety and Depression Scale (13 studies), Beck Anxiety Inventory, Generalized Anxiety Disorder-7 Scale, Depression Anxiety Stress Scale and Zung Self rating Anxiety Scale (3 studies each) The variation in prevalence rates of anxiety may also depend upon the stage of the HIV illness [21]. While newly diagnosed asymptomatic HIV patients feel socially stigmatized or are under excessive stress because of their HIV status others are concerned about the development of AIDS leading to anxiety [22].

Table 1. Prevalence rate of depression in patients with HIV

Location, Author	Assessed with	Sample size	Depression prevalence	Associated findings
Tanzania, Marwick and Kaaya [23]	CIS-R	220	15.5%	During HIV care, co-morbid psychiatric disorders should be identified and managed
Jamaica, Clarke et al. [24]	PHQ-9	63	43%	Age, sex, marital status, stress, living conditions, ART, & CD4+ count not associated with depression
Brazil, Campos et al.[25]	HADS	293	5.8%	
India, Khan [26]	BDI	82	30%	All subjects were under moderate levels of stress
India, Sivasubramanian et al. [27]	M.I.N.I.; DSM–IV	150	29%	Depression associated with low self-esteem and low social support
India, Nebhini et al. [28]	GHQ, SCID-CV	100	MDD 19%	
Malaysia, Hasanah et al. [29]	HADS	271	29.5%	Those who acquired the HIV infection via a heterosexual route had significantly lower social well-being compared to those who acquired HIV via drug injection
Albania, Morrison et al. [30]	Semi-structured interview	79	62.3%	Depression significantly associated with anxiety, greater number of barriers to care, and greater medical and social needs

Location, Author	Assessed with	Sample size	Depression prevalence	Associated findings
USA, Bhatia et al. [31]	CES-D	180	67%	Depression significantly associated female gender, low income, history of psychoactive substance abuse, and low access to medical care
Uganda, Kinyanda et al. [32]	M.I.N.I.	618	8.1%	Depression associated with psychosocial impairment, adverse life events, PTSD, GAD, and past history of deliberate self-harm
India, Agarwal et al. [33]	HADS	50	30%	46% of PLHA had low psychological well-being
South Africa, Pappin et al. [34]	HADS	716	25.4%	Depression was associated with stigma
Cameroon, L'akoa et al. [35]	PHQ-9	100	63%	Newly diagnosed HIV+ patients had higher prevalence of depression, severe immunosuppression, and harmful use of alcohol associated with depression
People's Republic of China, Su et al. [36]	BDI	258	71.9%	Depression was associated with less income and high perceived stress
India, Talukdar et al. [37]	BDI	175	56%	Poor QoL was associated with depression and high neuroticism score
Nigeria, Olagunju et al. [38]	SCID-NP	295	14.9%	Compared to the general population, PLHA suffer from more psychiatric disorders
South Korea, Song et al. [39]	BDI	82	21%	Depression was associated with poor adherence and anxiety. Comorbidities and unemployment were risk factors for depression.
People's Republic of China, Liu et al. [40]	CES-D	320	66.3%	Depression and anxiety in PLHA could be reduced by high social support
India, Chauhan et al. [41]	HADS	100	39%	Asymptomatic PLHA had significantly higher prevalence of alcohol dependence, adjustment disorder, & sexual dysfunction compared to controls

Table 1. (Continued)

Location, Author	Assessed with	Sample size	Depression prevalence	Associated findings
Israel, Levy et al. [42]	PHQ-9	57	24%	Cognitive disturbances and psychiatric illnesses were common in asymptomatic PLHA, but were independent immunological status, viral load, or treatment received
South Africa, Nel and Kagee [43]	BDI II	101	40.4%	ART adherence significantly related to depression
Romania, Largu et al. [44]	BDI II	146	41% (moderate 14%; mild 27%)	PLHA were afraid (of death, reaction of others to the diagnosis), confused (in terms of diagnosis, mode of infection, the future), angry (against the source of infection, themselves, God), felt guilty and blamed themselves
Malawi, Kim et al. [45]	CDRS-R	562	18.9%	7.1% of PLHA had suicidal ideation
Germany, Kittner et al. [46]	HADS	80	30% (male) 47% (female)	Guilt for the HIV infection present in 36% of PLHA
India, Bhatia and Munjal [47]	CES-D	160 on ART	58.7%	Depression was associated with low family income, unemployment, low education, not married, migration, poor relations with spouse, poor social support, and visiting commercial sex workers
People's Republic of China, Sun et al. [48]	CES-D	772	73.1%	Depression associated with health status, perceived social support, job, and gender
People's Republic of China, Qiu et al. [49]	PHQ-9	370	40.3%	Depression associated with employment status, sexual orientation, resident status, emergence of HIVrelated symptoms, stress, and social support
USA, Glémaud et al. [50]	PRIME MD	96 Haitian females	49%	12.5% of subjects gave a history of abuse; 34% of subjects had PTSD

Location, Author	Assessed with	Sample size	Depression prevalence	Associated findings
Lowther et al. [51]	Systematic review	66 original studies	33.60%	Low- and middle-income countries had a higher prevalence of depression (41.36%) compared to high-income countries (25.81%)
Western Europe and Canada, Robertson et al. 5 (2014) [5]	HADS	2,863	15.7%	Depression significantly more common in females than males and in cART experienced vs.cART naïve patients
Arseniou et al. [52]	Systemic electronic search of pubmed	138 studies	18-81%	Depression associated with female sex, old age, past history of depression, symptomatic HIV disease, stigma, occupational disability, body image changes, isolation, and debilitation, Alterations of: brain morphology, functional neural networks, white matter structure; abnormal HPT axis feedback, Tat protein, somatostatin dysregulation, & tryptophan degradation
USA, Kosiba [53]	MINI	131	55% MDD	
South Korea, Kee et al. [54]	BDI	840	36%	Depression associated with persistent symptoms, alcohol & tobacco use, & marital status
Brazil, Nomoto et al. [55]	BDI	59	61%	Depression significantly associated with low income, low social class, and poor QoL
Denmark, Slot et al. [56]	BDI	212	35%	Depression associated with stress, poor health, dissatisfaction with life situation, ART non-adherence, and past history of alcohol abuse or psychiatric treatment

Table 1. (Continued)

Location, Author	Assessed with	Sample size	Depression prevalence	Associated findings
Ethiopia, Eshetu et al. [57]	PHQ9	416	38.94%	Depression was associated with being female, age, stage of disease, low income, perceived stigma and recent hospitalization
Nigeria, Onyebueke [58]	MINI	180	27.8%	Risk of suicide was 7.8%
USA, O'Cleirig [59]	Medical records	503	21.9%	Subjects were HIV+ gay/bisexual men
India, Ghosh et al. [60]	HADS	100 female sex workers	30%	Modified HADS used
Ethopia, Tesfaw et al. [61]	HADS	417	41.2%	Perceived HIV stigma, HIV Stage III, poor social support and poor medication adherence were associated with depression.
Malayasia, Radzniwan [62]	DASS	206	36.9%	Co-morbidity significantly increased the odds of having depression
Canada, Choi et al. [63]	CES-D or the KPDS	3816	28% (point prevalence)	Prospective cohort study; 25.08% had depression at baseline, 43% had a recurrent episode during 2 years follow-up.
Rwanda, Smith Fawzi et al. [64]	CES-D adapted for children	193 (10-17yrs)	26%	12% attempted DSH; ART nonadherence was significantly associated with conduct problems and depression
China, Niu et al. [65]	Systematic review	94 studies	60.64% (16%-100%)	In 12 studies; women (36.6%–94.5%) more likely to be depressed than men (37.9%–71.8%). HIV-positive subjects had higher prevalence of depression and more severe depressive symptoms (17 studies)
India, Wani & Sankar [66]	Anxiety, Depression and Stress Scale	100	26% moderate & 74% severe depression	Married patients have higher levels of anxiety, stress and depression than unmarried patients

Location, Author	Assessed with	Sample size	Depression prevalence	Associated findings
India, Algoodkar et al. [67]	ICD 10	100	30%	Female gender, lack of family support, and HIV-positive status of the spouse associated with depression
Cameroon, Kanmogne et al. [68]	BDI II	270	33.73%	Depression associated with female sex & low education
Sudan, Elbadawi [69]	HADS	362	63.1%	Depression commoner in women, illiterate, married/widowed, not receiving counseling,
Brazil, Betancur et al. poor adherence to HAART [70]	BDI II	47	59.5%	Depression was the main reason for not taking medication (46.8%)
India, Deshmukh et al. [71]	DASS	754	50%	Female, illiterate, unemployed & low QOL mor depressed
Nigeria, Egbe [72]	Depression module CIDI	1187	28.2% MDE	MDD significantly associated with having planned suicide & marital status. Prevalence of suicidal ideation was 2.9%, 2.3% for suicide attempts
China Tao et al. [73]	HADS	364 MSM	36%	Depression associated with earlier ART initiation
Ghana, Kwakye [74]	DASS	138	87%	Depression negatively correlated with CD4+ count
Kazakhstan, Terloyeva et al[75]	PHQ-9	564	9.9%	Depression associated with ART treatment, positive HCV status, and being unmarried
S Africa, Rane et al. [76]	PHQ-9	1482	33%	Severe depression was associated with delayed presentation
Pakisthan, Hafeez [77]	SSDS	168	44%	Depression more common on those not on treatment, females and having CD4<500
China Zhou et al. [78]	CDI, CERQ, MSPSS, CSDS	155 (8-18 yrs)	32.41%	Social desirability, perceived social support, and catastrophizing significantly predicted depression.
Nigeria, Adoti et al. [79]	DASS	424	39.6%	Female gender, illiteracy, being divorced/widowed, unemployed, low income and low CD4 count were associated with depression

Table 1. (Continued)

Location, Author	Assessed with	Sample size	Depression prevalence	Associated findings
Ethiopia, Wondatir [80]	PHQ-9	416	32.9%	Depression significantly associated with 30-39 age group, history of hospitalisation, poor adherence, family history and CD4 count <250.
Canada, Tymchuk et al. [81]	PHQ-9	265	45%	Low education, unemployment, diabetes, reduced adherence to ART, neurocognitive disorders, low HQoL, reduced sleep, and domestic violence were associated with depression
India Kavya [82]	BDI	169	69%	Depression associated with age at diagnosis and relationship status
China Liu et al. [83]	Burns Depression Checklist	220	40%	Depression positively associated with bad sleep quality, hostility, perceived discrimination, and ART side effects and negatively with family support
Tanzania, Ngocho et al. [85]	EPDS	200 pregnant PLHA	25%	Depression significantly associated with being single, food insecurity, and HIV shame
China, Niu et al.[86]	Observational cohort study; PHQ9	410	39.3%	Prevalence of depression reduced to 10.5% at follow-up; bisexuality, homo-sexual transmission, not on ART, non-disclosure, higher levels of HIV/AIDS-related stress, & lack of social support associated with significant symptoms of depression and anxiety.

Location, Author	Assessed with	Sample size	Depression prevalence	Associated findings
Ethopia, Duko et al. [87]	HADS	363	32%	Depression significantly associated with living alone, poor social support, and HIV-related stigma
Malawi, Harrington et al. [88]	EPDS	725	9.5%	Depression associated with a history of depression, intimate partner violence, having an unintended current pregnancy, being unmarried, or employed
Ethiopia, Gebrezgiabher [89]	PHQ-9	411	14.6%	Depression associated with nonadherence to ART, eating two meals per day or less, having side effect of ART, being in the WHO Stage II or above of HIV/AIDS, and living alone
Ethiopia, Abbebe et al. [90]	BDI II	507	35.5%	Depression associated with age 20 to 24 years, history of opportunistic infection, poor medication adherence, low social support, and stigma
Guinea, Camara et al.[91]	HADS	160	16.9%	Depression significantly associated with BMI ≤18 and not receiving ART

Abbreviations: AIDS, acquired immunodeficiency syndrome; ART, antiretroviral therapy; BDI, Beck Depression Inventory; CDI, Children's Depression Inventory; CDRS-R, Children's Depression Rating Scale Revised; CERQ, Cognitive Emotion Regulation Questionnaire; CES-D, Center for Epidemiologic Studies Depression Scale; CIDI Composite International Diagnostic Interview; CIS-R, Clinical Interview Schedule-Revised; CSDS Children's Social Desirability scale; DSM, Diagnostic and Statistical Manual of Mental Disorders; GAD, generalized anxiety disorder; HADS, Hospital Anxiety and Depression Scale; HCV hepatitis C virus;HIV, human immunodeficiency virus; HQoL health-related quality of life; ICD, International Classification of Diseases; KPDS, Kessler Psychological Distress Scale; MDE, major depressive episode; M.I.N.I., Mini International Neuropsychiatric Interview; MSM, men who have sex with men; MSPSS, Multidimensional Scale of Perceived Social Support; PHQ-9, Patient Health Questionnaire 9; PLHA, persons living with HIV/AIDS; PTSD, post-traumatic stress disorder; QoL, quality of life; SCID-NP, Structured Clinical Interview for DSM-IV non-patient; SRDS, Self-rating depression scale.

Table 2. Prevalence rate of anxiety in patients with HIV

Location, Author	Assessed with	Sample size	Anxiety prevalence	Associated findings
Tanzania, Marwick & Kaaya[23]	CISR	220		Mixed anxiety & depression 12.7%, specific phobia 3.2%, panic disorder 1.8%
Brazil, Campos et al. [25]	HADS	293	12.6%	Severe anxiety was a predictor of non-adherence to ART during follow-up period
India, Khan [26]	CA-Test	82	63%	All subjects were under moderate stress
India, Sivasubramanian et al. [27]	M.I.N.I.; DSM-IV	150	24%	Anxiety associated with low levels of social support
Albania, Morrison et al. [30]	Semi-structured interview	79	82.3%	Anxiety significantly associated with depression, first-line ART, recent HIV diagnosis, and greater medical and social needs
India, Nebhini [28]	GHQ, SCID-CV	100	1% panic disorder	
Malaysia, Hasanah [29]	HADS	271	29.2%	
Nigeria, Olagunju et al. [92]	SCAN	4,000	21.7%	Anxiety was associated with low family support, lack of employment, and being unmarried
Canada, Ivanova et al. [93]	HADS	361 HIV+ women of reproductive age	37%	Anxiety associated with stigma, ART, and worries about reproductive health
India, Agarwal et al. [33]	HADS	50	54%	46% of PLWHA had low psychological well-being
USA, Nurutdinova et al. [94]	ICD 9CM	9003 medical records	18%	18% of HIV+ veterans met criteria for an anxiety disorder
USA, Reif et al. [95]	BSI, SF-12	40	33%	
USA, Lopes et al. [96]	AUDADIS-IV	149	33.43% men; 23.74% women	HIV + men four times as likely to meet criteria for an anxiety disorder compared to HIV− men (O.R.4.02), while HIV+ women were marginally more likely to meet criteria for an anxiety disorder compared to HIV− women (O.R. 1.17)

Location, Author	Assessed with	Sample size	Anxiety prevalence	Associated findings
India, Chauhan et al. [41]	HADS	100	19%	Asymptomatic PLWHA had significantly higher prevalence of alcohol dependence, adjustment disorder, and sexual dysfunction
Italy, Celesia et al. [97]	ZSRAS	251	47%	Anxiety was associated with a high number of ART switches
Nigeria, Olagunju et al.[38]	SCID-NP	295	8.1%	PLWHA suffer from more psychiatric disorders
USA, Parhami et al. [98]	Medical records of HIV + persons	7,834	16%	53% of the patients had a psychiatric condition, including mood disorder (23%) and substance-related disorder (19%)
China, Liu et al. [40]	ZSRAS	320	45.6%	Depression and anxiety in PLWHA could be reduced by high social support
Israel, Levy [42]	STAI	57	18%	Neurocognitive disturbances and psychiatric illnesses are common in asymptomatic PLWHA, independent of the time of being positive, immunological status, viral load, or treatment received
South Africa, Nel & Kagee [43]	BAI	101	28.7%	–
Romania, Largu et al. [44]	HAS	146	71% (54% mild, 14% severe, and 3% very severe anxiety)	PLWHA were afraid (of death, complications, other people's reaction to the diagnosis), confused (in terms of diagnosis, the mode of infection, the future), angry (against the source of infection, themselves, God), & felt guilty.
Germany, Kittner et al. [46]	HADS	80	40% (male) and 73% (female)	Guilt for the HIV infection was present in 36% of PLWHA
People's Republic of China, Sun et al. [48]	ZSRAS	772	49%	Anxiety associated with health status, social support, alcohol use, and condom use at the last sexual contact

Table 2. (Continued)

Location, Author	Assessed with	Sample size	Anxiety prevalence	Associated findings
People's Republic of China, Qiu et al. [49]	GAD-7	370	30.5%	Anxiety associated with employment status, sexual orientation, resident status, emergence of HIV-related symptoms, and stress
Ethiopia, Belete et al. [22]	BAI	436	22.2%	Being female, perceived stigma, started ART, and divorced were significantly associated with anxiety
Haitian females in USA, Glémaud et al. [50]	PRIME MD	96	42.7%	12.5% of subjects gave a history of abuse; 2.1% panic disorder;
S Africa, Breur et al. [99]	SAMISS, MINI	366	3%	
USA, Kosiba 2014 [53]	MINI	131		29% PD, 14.5% GAD, 22.9% SAA
Lowther et al. [53, 51]	Systematic review	66 original studies	28.38%	Low- and middle-income countries had a higher prevalence (33.92%) compared to high-income countries (25.53%)
South Korea, Kee et al. [54, 54]	STAI	840	32%	Anxiety associated with persistent symptoms, substance use and marital status
India, Ghosh et al. [60]	HADS	100	44%	Modified HADS used, female sex workers
Ethopia, Tesfaw et al. [61]	HADS	417	32.4%	Being female, divorced, co morbid TB and perceived HIV stigma associated with anxiety.
Malayasia, Radzniwan [62]	DASS	206	45.1%	
China, Niu et al. [65]	Systematic review	94 studies	43.13%(11.11% to 97.53%,)	Women (47%–80%) more likely to report anxiety than men (41.3%–58.6%). PLWHA more likely to experience anxiety
India Shukla et al. [100]	HAM-A	179 PLWHA on ART	7.7%	Anxiety associated with educational status, side-effects and duration of treatment.
Brazil, Betancur et al. [70]	BAI	47	44.7%	44.7% had moderate to severe anxiety

Location, Author	Assessed with	Sample size	Anxiety prevalence	Associated findings
China Tao et al. [73]	HADS	364 MSM	42%	Anxiety associated with earlier ART initiation
Ghana, Kwakye [74]	DASS	138	78.3%	Anxiety correlated negatively with CD4+ cell count of participants
S Africa, Rane et al. [76]	GAD-7	1482	9%	Anxiety associated with delayed presentation
Nigeria, Adoti et al. [79]	DASS	424	32.6%	Anxiety associated with lower age, female gender, low income, and low CD4 count
Pakisthan, Hafeez [77]	SAS	168	27.9%	Depression more common in those with CD4<500
India Kavya [82]	HAM-A	169	82%	
Tanzania, Ngocho et al. [85]	BSI	200 pregnant PLWHAS	23.5%	Anxiety was associated with being single, HIV shame and lifetime experience of violence.
China, Niu et al. [86]	observational cohort study; GAD-7	410	30.2%	Prevalence of anxiety dropped to 6.1% at follow-up; homosexual transmission, not on ART, non-disclosure, higher levels of stress, and lack of social support were associated with significant symptoms of anxiety.
Guinea, Camara et al. [91]	HADS	160	13.8%	Anxiety significantly associated with Age ≤40 yrs

Abbreviations: AIDS, Acquired immunodeficiency syndrome; ART, Antiretroviral therapy; AUDADIS-IV Alcohol Use Disorder and Associated Disabilities Interview Schedule – DSMIV Version; BAI, Beck Anxiety Inventory; BSI, Brief Symptom Index; CISR, Clinical Interview Schedule-Revised; (CA-Test)comprehensive Anxiety Test; DASS Depression anxiety stress scale; DSM, Diagnostic and Statistical Manual of Mental Disorders; GAD-7, Generalized Anxiety Disorder Scale; HADS, Hospital Anxiety and Depression Scale; HAS, Hamilton Anxiety Scale; HIV, human immunodeficiency virus; ICD, International Classification of Diseases; M.I.N.I., Mini-International Neuropsychiatric Interview; PLWHA, Persons living with HIV/AIDS; PRIME-MD Primary Care Evaluation of Mental Disorders Patient Health Questionnaire; PTSD, post-traumatic stress disorder; QoL, quality of life; SAMISS Substance and Mental Illness Symptom Screener; SCAN, Schedule for clinical assessment in neuropsychiatry; SCID Structured clinical interview for DSM; SCID-CV Structured Clinical Interview for the DSM-IV Clinician Version; SF-12 Short Form-12 mental health index; ZSRAS Zungsfelt rating anxiety scale.

Risk Factors Associated with Depression among HIV Patients

The confirmation of diagnosis of HIV is associated with profound changes in the subjects' life. In the weeks, months, and even years following this individual experiences a plethora of emotional reactions including anger, shock, sadness, denial and even depression. Studies indicate that the prevalence and severity of depression in PLWHA is associated with various factors, including inability to accept their disease status, symptoms related to HIV infection, substance use disorders, stigma, stress, fear of being ostracized or victimized, lower education, loss of job, lower socioeconomic status, disturbances in body image, migration, death of family members, unmarried status, poor relationship with spouse, and frequenting commercial sex workers [4, 24, 47, 55, 101, 102]. A study of 212 PLWHA from Denmark identified the following predictors of depression: stress, poor health, and dissatisfaction with life situation, belief that all aspects of life are affected by HIV infection, ART nonadherence, and past history of alcohol abuse or of psychiatric treatment [56].

Stage of Illness

Distinct from the stages of HIV/AIDS there are various stages of disease progression in the HIV/AIDS care continuum: confirmation of diagnosis, contact with HIV medical caregiver, undergoing treatment, at the beginning of ART, and during adherence to ART. Due to absence of physical symptoms the asymptomatic stage of HIV infection is psychologically the least distressing. A study on hospitalized asymptomatic HIV patients found relatively low prevalence of only 6% for depression and 7% for anxiety. However, the study also found significantly increased prevalence of adjustment disorder, alcohol dependence, and sexual dysfunction in PLWHA as compared to the normal population. With further progression of the HIV infection and gradual decline in $CD4^+$

cell count, the prevalence of psychological distress and psychiatric disorders also increase [103, 104].

Gender of the Patients

Differences in biological sex with regard to psychiatric disorders in PLWHA was studied in a large (nationally representative sample of 34,653 US adults), prospective, cross-sectional study. HIV-positive men were significantly more likely compared with HIV negative men to have a mood disorder, major depressive disorder or dysthymia, followed by any anxiety disorder, and lastly any personality disorder. On the other hand HIV-positive women did not have an elevated prevalence of psychiatric disorders [96]. More recent studies have revealed various direct and indirect factors linked to the susceptibility of females to HIV transmission. The problem is further compounded due to the fact that females in developing countries have low levels of education, health, and hygiene. One study from Bangladesh reported that female sex workers were unable to convince their sexual partner to have safe sex [105]. The prevalence of depression in females is higher than in males in the general population as well as among HIV patients with injectable drug use [106]. Gender differences have also been observed in the manifestations of depression. Somatic symptoms of anxiety, easy fatigability, hypochondriac symptoms, poor appetite, and insomnia are reported more frequently by depressed women [107, 108, 109]. It is obvious that depression rating across the genders will vary depending on the presence or absence of these items in a rating scale. While two studies addressing the gender and psychiatric disorders in PLWHA observed that females had higher levels of anxiety and depression compared to males [110, 111] opposite findings were also reported by two studies [96, 112]. However, the majority of Indian studies have found that women have higher rates of depression and anxiety compared to men [113, 114]. The relation between the patients' gender and prevalence of anxiety and depression in PLWHA therefore needs further detailed evaluation.

DEPRESSION AND HIV INFECTION

In PLWHA prior history of mood disorders depression may occur due to infection of CNS by HIV. On the other hand, psychosocial factors like stigma, stress, fear of being ostracized or victimized may precipitate an episode or relapse of depression in an individual newly diagnosed as HIV-positive [115]. The findings of a two year longitudinal study revealed that in the intermediate term symptomatic HIV disease but not by HIV infection increases the risk of depression. However, a past history of depression or having two or more psychiatric disorders was strong predictors of future vulnerability to depression [116].

The 1996–1997 HIV Cost and Services Utilization Study (HCSUS) was a nationally representative study of psychiatric disorders among adult PLWHA in the US. Utilizing the Composite International Diagnostic Interview (CIDI) the 12-month prevalence of any psychiatric disorder was 32.8% including major depression (22%); dysthymia (5%); generalized anxiety disorder (4.1%); and panic disorder (15.5%) [117]. A multisite cohort of 1027 women living with HIV in the US used the WHO's CIDI to evaluate the prevalence, comorbidity, and correlates of 12-month psychiatric disorders. Results showed that 53.9% had at least one 12-month disorder. Mood disorder prevalence was 22.1% compared to 10.8% in the general women's population. The most common mood disorder was major depressive disorder (20.0%) [118].

A study of patients with history of deliberate self-harm (DSH) following recent HIV diagnosis revealed that the diagnosis of HIV increased the risk of DSH by 16%. Younger age, female gender, and psychiatric diagnoses further increased the risk of DSH. Patients blamed some stressors associated with HIV for the DSH, especially absence of psychosocial and health support, fear of being detested or persecuted, and fear of adverse impact on psychological, social, economic and health statuses [119]. A systematic review of mental health of PLWHA in China revealed that the prevalence of suicidal ideation in the past year ranged from 29.5% to 34.1%. The prevalence of attempted suicide in the past year varied from 3.8% to 8%. There was no significant gender difference observed [65].

ANXIETY AND HIV INFECTION

Anxiety is experienced by PLWHA at the time of initial detection, onset of symptoms, and progression of HIV infection. An early study reported that even though symptoms of anxiety were commonly seen in HIV positive individuals, but the prevalence of syndromal anxiety disorders is not significantly higher than in non-HIV positive individuals [120]. However, more recent studies report that that the prevalence of anxiety and depression in PLWHA is significantly higher than their prevalence in the general population [54]. Both anxiety and HIV have common etiological factors including alcohol and substance abuse, males having a bisexual relationship and males having sex with males [121]. Studies indicate that anxiety in PLWHA is associated with a past history of smoking, concurrent substance use disorder, confirmation of HIV positive status within the past year, persistent symptoms presenting for >7 days in the past 6 months [54], pain, minimum family support, and the spouse having AIDS [122]. An Indian study reported the prevalence of anxiety disorders (most commonly generalized anxiety disorder) in 36% PLWHA, which was higher than that found in studies conducted in developed countries [122].

In the HCSUS 12-month prevalence of GAD was 4.1%; and 15.5% for panic disorder [117]. A multisite cohort of 1027 women living with HIV in the US evaluated with CIDI revealed the prevalence of Anxiety disorder in women living with HIV was 45.4% compared to 23.2% in the general population, The most common anxiety disorders were specific phobias (22.1%), social phobia (13.9%), Panic disorder (PD) (6.27%) and generalized anxiety disorder (GAD) (5.28%) [118].

GAD and PD were detected in 15.8% and 10.5% of HIV seropositive persons versus 2.1% and 2.5% of the general population, respectively [123, 124, 125, 126]. In a few studies of HIV positive patients the prevalence of

PD has ranged from 11% to 16% [4, 127, 128, 129]. In PLWHA with resolved grief the prevalence of PD is less as compared to those with unresolved grief [130]. In various studies on PLWHA the prevalence of GAD varied from 6.5% to 20% [4, 128, 129, 131, 132, 133]. Studies indicate that with the passage after the initial diagnosis there was a significant reduction in the prevalence of GAD [130]. In one study 9% of 190 PLWHA suffered from simple phobia [131].

YOUTHS WITH HIV/AIDS

Youths with HIV/AIDS are reported to have high rates of depression which is up to four times higher than that in the general adolescent population [134, 135]. Anxiety disorders including phobias, separation anxiety, agoraphobia, GAD, and PD are not uncommon in children and adolescents with HIV/AIDS [136]. Symptoms of adolescent depression are similar to that in adults. However, depressive symptoms including loss of appetite or fatigue are difficult to differentiate from symptoms of the medical illness and side effects of HIV medications [137]. Young people with HIV/AIDS suffering from depression or anxiety, due to increased high-risk sexual behaviors, have an increased risk of acquiring other sexually transmitted diseases or becoming pregnant [138]. Untreated depression in youths with HIV/AIDS may negatively affect markers of HIV progression including CD4 counts and viral loads [139]. Pharmacotherapy of depression and anxiety in children and adolescents is usually with SSRIs. However, in view of reports of increased risk of suicidality in children and adolescents on SSRIs, they should be closely monitored. TCAs can be sedating and toxic in overdose and are less commonly used. Further, the metabolism of TCAs is inhibited by the HIV drug Ritonavir thereby increasing its potential for toxicity [140]. Depression is associated with decreased adherence to ART and effective treatment of depression may improve adherence and overall outcomes for HIV-infected youth [141, 142].

IMPACT OF HIV/AIDS

In view of the finding that PLWHA suffer from psychiatric symptoms and disorders more frequently than the general population, it is considered that HIV infection and psychiatric disorders are significant related risk factors. On the other hand, HIV infection occurs more often than in the general population in people with a major psychiatric disorder. Studies indicate that symptomatic HIV disease and past history of psychiatric disorders, but not asymptomatic HIV disease, are predictors of vulnerability for depression [116]. Studies indicate a bidirectional association consisting of complex biological and psychosocial interaction between depression and HIV disease [143]. This leads us to two questions: 1) why does HIV infection result in depression and anxiety; and 2) what are the effects of depression and anxiety on HIV infection.

HIV INFECTION RESULTING IN DEPRESSION AND ANXIETY

Various factors claimed to be the cause of depression and anxieties among PLWHA have been identified across studies. These can be grouped as psychosocial and biological factors causing depression and anxiety among patients with HIV. The initial diagnosis of HIV is immediately followed by psychological distress in the individual. It was expected that Adjustment problems would be commonly detected among newly diagnosed HIV patients [144]. However, one study that looked into this aspect reported that ~71% of patients were depressed for longer periods than the criterion for adjustment disorder [145]. The progression of HIV disease is clearly associated with increased depression [146, 147].

Stigma

HIV/AIDS remains a highly stigmatizing illness and is present frequently, rather invariably, in PLWHA. Studies have repeatedly found that stigma of HIV/AIDS is correlated with anxiety, depression, and other psychosocial problems [148, 149, 150, 151]. Patients with a highly stigmatizing illness like HIV/AIDS are well aware about how other people perceive them because of their condition. This is termed as perceived stigma [152]. Stigmatization results in restriction in social activities, and because of their status, they may begin to agree with the negative stereotypes linked with their condition. This process is termed as internalized stigma [153]. Internalized stigma may result in psychosocial distress, anxiety, and depression [147, 154, 155]. High levels of stigma has been associated with increased levels of anxiety and depression [150], poor utilization of HIV voluntary counseling and testing services [156], delay in seeking HIV/AIDS treatment [157], poor retention in follow-up [158], poor ART adherence [159], and increased risky behavior like unsafe sex practices [154].

Biological Model

The biological relationship between anxiety, depression and HIV has generated increasing interest and research in the past three decades since it may have therapeutic implications [160]. It has also been suggested that biological mechanisms may cause anxiety and depression in PLWHA [161]. Depression may, by several direct and indirect mechanisms, affect the progression of HIV infection. The neurotransmitter serotonin plays a role in both depression and immunity and therefore has been studied as a direct mediator of the process. In the body, serotonin controls the immune cell's production of additional receptors and signaling molecules and thereby increases the body's production of the types of immune cells responsible for effectively combating the infection by destroying infected cells. Serotonin also reduces HIV reproduction within the infected cell

[162]. Research has also reported that antidepressant medications by increasing serotonin levels may augment the body's ability to destroy HIV through actions on key immune cells [163]. HIV infection may predispose PLWHA to depression by several interrelated mechanisms including increasing cytokines through activation of microglia and astrocytes; increasing neurotoxicity, especially in dopaminergic neurons; along with reduction in brain-derived neurotrophic factor and monoaminergic function. These viral pathways interact with psychosocial factors to create the depressive state [164]. On the other hand depression-related increases in cortisol and other stress related hormones, may cause poor immune function by blunting and dysregulating the response of immune cells and their infection-fighting products, as well as increasing HIV replication [165]. Systemic immune dysregulation is also associated with anxiety and depression [165].

In addition, biopsychosocial factors in depression, including increased hopelessness, decreased social support, decreased medication adherence, increased substance abuse, and increased risk taking behaviors with probability of contracting additional sexually transmitted diseases, play an essential role through some of the same central mediators. The combined effect of these factors leads to measurably worse outcomes for patients, specifically increased disability, faster progression to AIDS, and decreased lifespan. It is imperative for the mental health professional to look for these contributing factors, as each of them is amenable to therapy with resultant improvement in immune outcome. Studies have proved that reduction in depressive symptoms improve immune cell function, increases immune cell counts and decreases viral load [167].

Effects of Depression and Anxiety on HIV Infection

Depression causes various direct and indirect morbidities, which include suicidal behavior [168], increased use of health care facilities [169], and poor QoL [129]. It is important to identify depression among PLWHA, as depression is associated with increased chances of HIV transmission [170] and ART nonadherence [171, 172, 173], resulting in failure to suppress viral load [174] and increased HIV disease progression [175, 176, 177, 178]. There are other mechanisms caused by depression that lead to a faster progression of HIV infection to AIDS, such as elevated cortisol secretion [15] and HIV replication through an increase in norepinephrine secretion [179]. Even AIDS-related death, specifically in females, was associated with chronic depression [104, 180].

Depression and Disease Progression

HIV disease progression has changed significantly since the introduction of highly active ART (HAART). A good outcome depends on the patient's adherence to the medication regimen. Depression in PLWHA is associated with nonadherence to ART, which adversely affects the outcome of HIV disease [181, 182, 183]. It has been observed that baseline depression does not influence ART adherence; but it is affected by depression occurring during the treatment period [184]. Treatment of depression in PLWHA with antidepressants is associated with a reduction in symptoms of depression, better adherence to their ART and improved laboratory parameters [185, 186].

Effects of Antiretroviral Drugs

A systematic review of the relevant literature revealed that PLWHA on ART have a higher prevalence of anxiety and depression as compared to non-HIV positive population [51]. As a result, depression and anxiety was partly attributed to antiretroviral medications. On the other hand a longitudinal study of anxiety, depression, stress and QOL in PLWHA revealed that ART improved mental health status and QOL, irrespective of the treatment strategy i.e., CD4 guided scheduled treatment interruption (STI) compared to continuous treatment (CT) [187]. On the other hand few studies have reported that depression and anxiety attributed to antiretroviral drugs (mainly efavirenz) showed significant improvement on substitution with another drug (e.g., nevirapine) [188, 189].

MANAGEMENT OF DEPRESSION AND ANXIETY IN HIV POSITIVE SUBJECTS

Management of depression and anxiety in PLWHA is based on the twin principles of pharmacotherapy and psychotherapy. It must be emphasized that subsyndromal presentation of anxiety and depression is also associated with adverse health outcomes and poor self-care in PLWHA. Therefore, it is imperative to treat subsyndromal disorders [174]. Apart from symptomatic relief the management of comorbid depression and anxiety improves the QOL of PLWHA also improves ART adherence [190, 191]. Improved ART adherence may, in turn, reduce symptoms of depression [192].

PHARMACOLOGICAL INTERVENTION

In general, pharmacotherapy of depression in PLWHA does not differ fundamentally from treatment of depression in other patients. Various studies have proved that antidepressants are efficacious in treating depression in PLWHA [193, 194]. Therefore antidepressants should invariably be a part of the therapeutic regimen. The aim of treatment is the complete remission of symptoms of depression. The treatment of depression in PLWHA should comprise of acute phase therapy, maintenance phase therapy and prophylaxis of a relapse which should be continued for at least six months. On completion of treatment antidepressant medication should be tapered gradually over a period of weeks. After starting antidepressant medication benefits are experienced after two weeks, but side effects may occur much earlier. Patients need to be aware of this. A non-response to medication is considered when the standard dose of the antidepressant does not give relief to the patient after a period of four to six weeks. At this point a switch to an antidepressant of another class is recommended followed by a four week wait for therapeutic benefits. Alternatively, augmentation with lithium or thyroid preparations may be considered. At times the combination of two antidepressants might be useful. While choosing an antidepressant keep in mind the side effect profile and match it with the patient's symptoms.

A review of psychopharmacotherapy in PLWHA observed a paucity of studies carried out after the introduction of currently used antiretroviral regimens; however, it was found that antidepressants and anxiolytics are widely used [195]. Antidepressants that were found to be useful in the treatment of depression in PLWHA include imipramine, desipramine, nortriptyline, amitriptyline, fluoxetine, sertraline, paroxetine, citalopram, escitalopram, fluvoxamine, venlafaxaine, nefazodone, trazodone, bupropion, and mirtazapine [196] and no drug is more efficacious than others [197]. Double-blind randomised control trials have been done with imipramine, fluoxetine, sertraline, and paroxetine [198].

In the management of anxiety in PLWHA it is recommended that psychopharmacotherapy should be avoided if psychotherapeutic modalities are available, especially in older patients because of greater chances of polypharmacy and increased risk for drug-drug interactions [199]. However, to support the older PLWHA's sense of control and autonomy it is helpful to initiate psychopharmacotherapy in low doses. Benzodiazepines (BZDs), the most common anxiolytic, are associated with side effects including sedation, amnesia and paradoxical reactions (disinhibition, confusion, etc.) [190], interaction with protease inhibitors and alcohol, and most importantly lead to dependence. Hence for long term treatment Selective serotonin re-uptake inhibitors (SSRIs) are the preferred medication. For short-term pharmacotherapy of anxiety, short-to intermediate-acting BZDs, like lorazepam and oxazepam which lack active metabolites, are recommended. However, for PLWHA receiving ART clonazepam and lorazepam are probably the BZDs of choice as they lack active metabolites and are safe in terms of drug–drug interactions [200, 201]. Buspirone is an alternative which is non-sedating, safe in overdose, and does not lead to dependence. The major drawback of buspirone is the delay in onset of action compared to immediate onset of action of BZDs. Moreover, as it is metabolized by CYP3A4 it should be avoided in PLWHA receiving protease inhibitors [191, 202]. Other anxiolytics with low abuse potential include hydroxyzine, diphenhydramine, pregabalin and the nutritional supplement, valerian. However hydroxyzine and diphenhydramine due to their anti-cholinergic side effects should be used with caution in older adults, while pregabalin is sedating. As hypnotics the non-BZDs (eszopiclone, zopiclone, zolpidem, and zaleplon) have comparatively low dependence potential and lack daytime sedation that may occur with BZDs. However these drugs are also metabolized by CYP3A4 and should be avoided in PLWHA receiving protease inhibitors [201, 203].

Selective Serotonin Reuptake Inhibitors

SSRIs are effective and well tolerated, and are the first line antidepressant medication in depressed PLWHA is more suitable than TCAs for long-term therapy [204]. The probability of adverse effects is reduced by initiating treatment with low doses. A few recent reports have blamed SSRI medication for precipitating suicide, especially in children and adolescents. However, a Swedish database study, involving analysis of nearly 15000 suicides found no increased risk for the treatment of depressed individuals with SSRIs [205]. Nonetheless, psychiatrists should closely monitor patients with psychiatric disorders, especially depression, for suicide risk regardless of their medication, and, if indicated, ask for suicidal thoughts or self-harm in order to institute appropriate treatment.

Fluoxetine produced significant reduction in depression compared to placebo [101]. Other SSRIs also produced significant reduction in depressive symptoms, but comparative effectiveness of various SSRIs has not been ascertained [191, 206]. All the SSRIs can be used in PLWHA [207, 208]. The most common side effects of SSRIs include anxiety, agitation, akathisia, weight loss, and sexual dysfunction [190]. Since the

SSRIs are metabolized by CYP450 isoenzymes [209] ARV medications may alter their plasma levels. In this regard sertraline, citalopram, and escitalopram are preferred due to their low drug interactions [206, 220]. However, when SSRIs are given to PLWHA who are on ART the chance of serotonin syndrome is increased [211].

Tricyclic Antidepressants

Tricyclic antidepressants (TCAs) are effective in PLWHA but side effects are more frequent reducing their acceptability. Due to their anticholinergic effects, they are contraindicated in patients with urinary retention and closed-angle glaucoma and should be avoided in patients with bundle branch blocks. Another major problem is that TCAs are easier to overdose than SSRIs.

Specific Issues with Newer Antidepressants

Nefazodone is an effective antidepressant in PLWHA [212]. However, in view of nefazodone-induced hepatitis, it should be used cautiously in PLWHA because of the frequent occurrence of viral hepatitis. Ritonavir, efavirenz, and nelfinavir interferes with the metabolism of bupropion [213, 214].

Psychostimulants

Psychostimulants have a role as adjuvant in the treatment of depression in PLWHA, especially in the presence of neglect of self-care and nutrition in advanced HIV patients [215, 216]. A randomized control trial of methylphenidate and desipramine in depressed PLWHA showed treatment response in 43% and 40% of subjects respectively [215]. A similar study observed treatment response in 73% of those assigned to dextroamphetamine [216].

Hormonal Therapies

In HIV infection reduced testosterone levels produces depression, anorexia, anergia, and sexual dysfunction. Hormonal therapies have been advocated to treat depression in PLWHA based on this hypothesis with some success [217]. Obviously this therapy can only be recommended in PLWHA with decreased testosterone level.

NONPHARMACOLOGICAL INTERVENTIONS

Nonpharmacological or Psychotherapeutic interventions beneficial for anxiety and depression in PLWHA include cognitive behavior therapy (CBT), interpersonal therapy (IPT), cognitive–behavioral-oriented group psychotherapy (CBGP), experiential group psychotherapy (EGT) and supportive psychotherapy. Important elements of psychotherapy for PLWHA include dealing with stigma, punishment beliefs, discrimination, and reducing barriers to adherence to both ART and psychopharmacological drugs. Other psychotherpeutic approaches that appear to be useful include cognitive–behavioral stress management (CBSM), stress management interventions, mindfulness-based intervention (MBI), guided imagery, progressive muscular relaxation training, self-hypnosis, biofeedback, and aerobic and resistance exercise.[194]

Cognitive Behavior Therapy

The efficacy of CBT in treating anxiety and depression in PLWHA is attested by randomized controlled studies, meta-analysis, and systematic analysis [218, 219, 220]. While evaluating the feasibility and effectiveness of group CBT in combination with medication in 13 depressed PLWHA, Lee et al. [218] observed a significant improvement in depression. They found that cognitive restructuring was the most helpful psychotherapeutic process of CBT. A meta-analysis of 15 randomized controlled trials of CBT in depressed PLWHA reported significant improvement in symptoms of depression ($d=0.33$), anxiety ($d=0.30$), anger ($d=1.00$), and stress ($d=0.43$) [219]. Another systemic review involving 2,173 participants from 20 studies showed that CBT was effective in the treatment of depression and anxiety in PLWHA, with effect sizes ranging from 0.02 to 1.02 for depression and 0.04 to 0.70 for anxiety [220].

Interpersonal Therapy

A randomized clinical trial of IPT versus supportive psychotherapy for treatment of depression in PLWHA reported that both treatments resulted in significantly lower scores on the Hamilton Rating Scale for Depression (HAM-D) and the Beck Depression Inventory (BDI). However a differential improvement for IPT was observed by mid treatment and persisted at termination. This indicated that IPT has advantages over supportive psychotherapy [221]. Another randomized controlled trial involved 101 depressed PLWHA with score ≥15 on the HAM-D found that IPT and supportive psychotherapy plus imipramine produced a significantly greater reduction in HAM-D scores compared to CBT and supportive psychotherapy without imipramine [222].

Supportive Psychotherapy

The focus of supportive psychotherapy is to strengthen mental functions that are acutely or chronically inadequate to meet the demands of the external world. Supportive psychotherapy in PLWHA is primarily based on teaching coping skills. A randomized clinical trial of IPT and supportive psychotherapy reported clinically significant reduction in depression in both groups, which were maintained at follow-up after 3 months. An additional important finding was that the occurrence of unprotected anal intercourse was reduced after supportive therapy [221].

Cognitive-Behavioral-Oriented Group Psychotherapy

The efficacy of CBGP program in improving psychosocial adjustment to HIV infection was evaluated in 47 completing patients. A significant improvement was found in Psychosocial Adjustment to Illness Scale scores, health care orientation, vocational environment, domestic environment, sexual relation, social environment, and extended family relationships [223].A randomized control study evaluated the effectiveness of CBGP and EGT against waiting-list control group (WCG). Both psychotherapeutic interventions reduced psychological distress significantly compared to the WCG [224].A systematic review of four randomized controlled trials of CBGP for depression in PLWHA revealed that CBGP was an effective intervention for reducing depressive symptoms in PLWHA in comparison to waiting list controls [225].

Experiential Group Psychotherapy

A randomized control study compared the effects of EGT and CBGP on asymptomatic homosexual PLWHA versus WCG. Results revealed that both therapies reduced psychological distress, but there was no significant difference between the two therapies. In addition no significant changes were observed in the intervention groups as compared with the WCG in coping styles, emotional expression, and social support [224].

Cognitive–Behavioral Stress Management

CBSM intervention is a promising approach to facilitate positive adjustment in PLWHA. A review of 21 CBSM intervention studies designed to enhance the ability to effectively cope with a wide variety of life stressors in PLWHA gave the following findings: Positive changes in perceived stress, depression, anxiety, global psychological functioning, QOL and social support was reported by most of the studies. However, for coping and health status outcomes the results were mixed [226]. CBSM training of PLWHA on cART reduces depression and anxiety [226, 227], improves QOL [226, 227] and global psychological functioning [228] but does not improve adherence to ART or surrogate markers of HIV-1 [227].

Stress Management Interventions

A meta-analysis of 35 randomized controlled trials examining the efficacy of 46 separate stress-management interventions for 3077 PLWHA, revealed that compared to control subjects stress management interventions significantly improved anxiety, depression, distress, fatigue, and QoL, but had no effect on immunological ($CD4^+$ counts and viral load) or hormonal functions [229]. A recent study concluded that, both group stress management and group CBT were effective in reducing depression, anxiety and perceived stress in PLWHA. However, the former was more effective than the latter in reducing depression, anxiety and perceived stress in PLWHA [230].

Mindfulness-Based Therapy

MBIs to mitigate stress among PLHWA has attracted increasing attention. A meta-analysis was performed of 16 studies of MBI involving 1059 PLWHA for an average of 8 years with 65% on ART. Analysis revealed significant reduction in anxiety and depression with improved

QOL among MBI participants compared to control subjects. There was no significant change in immunological outcomes (i.e., CD4 counts) [231].

Aerobic and Resistance Exercise

In addition to the beneficial physiological changes, exercise also reduces depression and anxiety in PLWHA. One investigation using aerobic exercise as the primary intervention for HIV-associated depressive symptoms found that 60 minutes of moderate intensity aerobic exercise conducted 3 days a week is associated with reductions in depressive symptoms and/or significant improvements in QOL [232]. Similar findings have been reported in other studies [233, 234]. A review of 24 RCTs was carried out to understand the health benefits of aerobic, resistance, and combined aerobic/resistance training among PLWHA and its effects on immune status. Studies have consistently shown physiological improvements across clinical measurements of health such as BMI, waist circumference, blood lipids, muscular strength, and cardiorespiratory fitness. The review found no effect on immunological measured variables regardless of exercise intensity [235].

Effects of Psychosocial Interventions

A systematic review and meta-analysis of 62 studies investigated the effectiveness of different psychosocial treatments for PLWH and mental health problems. The overall effect of psychosocial interventions on mental health outcomes was Hedges' $\hat{g} = 0.19$, 95% CI [0.13, 0.25], p\0.001. Thus, compared to a control condition psychotherapeutic interventions may have a positive effect on mental health. However, the effect size was small. The overall effect of psychosocial interventions on mental health shows that the pooled effect sizes for depression and psychological well-being were larger ($\hat{g} = 0.21$ and 0.20) than those for anxiety and quality of life ($\hat{g} = 0.09$ and 0.13). The meta-analysis found that, overall, psychosocial interventions may have a small positive effect on the mental health of PLWH. No differences in effect were found between the three intervention type, which means that symptom-oriented interventions, supportive interventions, and meditation may all be effective. A larger improvement in depression may be obtained when only participants with depressive symptoms are included in the study; when interventions are provided by psychologists; when treatment duration is 12–18 h; and when the intervention is focused on improving mental health [236].

CONCLUSION

Depression and anxiety occurs more frequently in people living with HIV/AIDS (PLWHA) than in the general population. The prevalence of depression and anxiety in PLWHA is reported to vary from 5.8% to 87% and 3% to 82.3%, respectively. The coexistence of these disorders has a major impact on PLWHA. Anxiety and depression increase the morbidity of HIV by poor adherence to treatment, increased risk for suicide, greater chance for recurrence and various other significant mechanisms. Studies indicate that effective management of anxiety and depression in PLWHA results in improved antiretroviral adherence, improved quality of life and increased survival. The management of anxiety and depression in PLWHA involves both pharmacological and nonpharmacological therapies. Benzodiazepines are only indicated for short periods of time. Clonazepam and lorazepam may be preferred due to lack of active metabolites and less drug–drug interactions. SSRIs are the preferred antidepressants. Though the different SSRIs are equally effective, sertraline, citalopram, and escitalopram are preferred in PLWHA to avoid interactions with antiretrovirals. Various psychotherapeutic interventions, including supportive psychotherapy, cognitive behavior therapy, interpersonal therapy, cognitive–behavioral-oriented group psychotherapy, experiential group psychotherapy, cognitive–behavioral stress management, stress management interventions, cognitive remediation, mindfulness-based therapy, and aerobic and resistance exercise have all been found to be useful in treating depression and anxiety in PLWHA. However, the comparative efficacy of the different nonpharmacological intervention for the management of anxiety and depression in PLWHA is yet to be determined.

ACKNOWLEDGMENT

This chapter is based partly on the work done for the article: Chaudhury Suprakash, BakhlaAjai K, and Saini Raji. Prevalence, impact, and management of depression and anxiety in HIV patients: A Review. Neurobehavioral HIV Medicine 2016;7: 15-30.

REFERENCES

[1] World Health Organization. (2007). *WHO Case Definitions of HIV for Surveillance and Revised Clinical Staging and Immunological Classification of HIV-Related Disease in Adults and Children.* Geneva: World Health Organization.

[2] World Health Organization. (2016). *Health Topics. HIV/AIDS Online.* Geneva, World Health Organization. Available from: http://www.who.int/topics/hiv_aids/en/. Accessed February 24, 2016.

[3] Bravo, P., Edwards, A., Rollnick, S., and Elwyn, G. (2010). Tough decisions faced by people living with HIV: a literature review of psychosocial problems. *AIDS Review* 12(2):76–88.

[4] Bing, E.G., Burnam, M.A., Longshore, D., Fleishman, J.A., Sherbourne, C.D., and London, A.S. (2001). Psychiatric disorders and drug use among human immunodeficiency virus-infected adults in the United States. *Archives of General Psychiatry* 58:721–28.

[5] Robertson, K., Bayon, C., Molina, J.M., McNamara, P., Resch, C., Muñoz-Moreno, J.A., and van Wyk, J. (2014). Screening for

neurocognitive impairment, depression, and anxiety in HIV-infected patients in Western Europe and Canada. *AIDS Care* 26(12):1555–61.

[6] Andrinopoulos, K., Clumm G., Murphy, D.A., Harper, G., Perez, L., Xu, J., Cunningham, S., Ellen, J.M., and Adolescent Medicine Trials Network for HIV/AIDS Interventions. (2011). Health related quality of life and psychosocial correlates among HIV-infected adolescent and young adult women in the US. *AIDS Education and Prevention* 23:367–81.

[7] Peter, E., Kamath, R., Andrews, T., and Hegde, B.M. (2014).Psychosocial determinants of health-related quality of life of people living with HIV/AIDS on antiretroviral therapy at Udupi District, Southern India. *International Journal of Preventive Medicine* 5(2):203–9.

[8] Reisner, S.L., Mimiaga, M.J., Skeer, M., Perkovich, B., Johnson, C.V., and Safren, S.A. (2009). A review of HIV antiretroviral adherence and intervention studies among HIV-infected youth. *Topics in HIV Medicine* 17(1):14–25.

[9] Psaros, C., O'Cleirigh, C., Bullis, J.R., Markowitz, S.M., and Safren, S.A. (2013). The influence of psychological variables on health-related quality of life among HIV-positive individuals with a history of intravenous drug use. *Journal of Psychoactive Drugs* 45(4):304–12.

[10] Sin, N.L., and DiMatteo, M.R. (2014). Depression treatment enhances adherence to antiretroviral therapy: a meta-analysis. *Annals of Behavioral Medicine* 47(3):259–69.

[11] Chipimo, P.J., and Fylkesnes, K. (2009). Mental distress in the general population in Zambia: Impact of HIV and social factors: *BMC Public Health* 9: 298. http:// www.ncbi.nlm.nih.gov/pmc/articles/PMC2744699.

[12] Chipimo, P.J., and Fylkesnes, K. (2013). Human Immunodeficiency Virus Infection and Co-Morbid Mental Distress. In *Current Perspectives in HIV Infection* edited by Shailendra K. Saxena, 125-136. Rijeka: Intech.

[13] Meade, C.S., and Sikkema, K.J. (2005). HIV risk behavior among adults with severe mental illness: a systematic review. *Clinical Psychology Review* 25(4):433–57.

[14] Simoni, J.M., Safren, S.A., Manhart, L.E., Lyda, K., Grossman, C.I., Rao, D., Mimiaga, M.J., Wong, F.Y., Catz, S.L., Blank, M.B., DiClemente, R., and Wilson, I.B. (2011). Challenges in addressing depression in HIV research: assessment, cultural context, and methods. *AIDS and Behavior* 15(2):376–88.

[15] Schuster, R., Bornovalova, M., Hunt, E. (2012). The influence of depression on the progression of HIV: direct and indirect effects. *Behaviour Modification* 36(2):123–45.

[16] Phillips, K.D., Sowell, R.L., Rojas, M., Tavakoli, A., Fulk, L.J., and Hand, G.A. (2004). Physiological and psychological correlates of fatigue in HIV disease. *Biological Research for Nursing* 6(1):59–74.

[17] Dubé, B., Benton, T., Cruess, D.G., and Evans, D.L. (2005). Neuropsychiatric manifestations of HIV infection and AIDS. *Journal of Psychiatry and Neuroscience* 30:237–46.

[18] Ciesla, J.A., and Roberts, J.E. (2001). Meta-analysis of the relationship between HIV infection and risk for depressive disorders. *American Journal of Psychiatry* 158:725–30.

[19] Rabkin, J.G. (2008). HIV and depression: 2008 review and update. *Current HIV/AIDS Report* 5(4):163–71.

[20] Willard, S., Holzemer, W.L., Wantland, D.J., Cuca, Y.P., Kirksey, K.M., Portillo, C.J., Corless, I.B., Rivero-Méndez, M., Rosa, M.E., Nicholas, P.K., Hamilton, M.J., Sefcik, E., Kemppainen, J., Canaval, G., Robinson, L., Moezzi, S., Human, S., Arudo, J., Eller, L.S., Bunch, E., Dole, P.J., Coleman, C., Nokes, K., Reynolds, N.R., Tsai, Y.F., Maryland, M., Voss, J., and Lindgren, T. (2009). Does "asymptomatic" mean without symptoms for those living with HIV infection? *AIDS Care* 21(3):322–8.

[21] Perkins, D.O., Stern, R.A., Golden, R.N., Murphy, C., Naftolowitz, D., and Evans, D.L. (1994). Mood disorders in HIV infection. Prevalence and risk factors in a non epicenter of the AIDS epidemic. *American Journal of Psychiatry* 15:233–6.

[22] Belete, A., Andaregie, G., Tareke, M., Birhan, T., and Azale, T. (2014). Prevalence of anxiety and associated factors among people living with HIV/AIDS at Debretabor general hospital anti retro viral clinic Debretabor, Amhara, Ethiopia, 2014. *American Journal of Psychiatry and Neuroscience* 2(6):109–14.

[23] Marwick, K.F., and Kaaya, S.F. (2010). Prevalence of depression and anxiety disorders in HIV-positive outpatients in rural Tanzania. *AIDS Care* 22(4):415–9.

[24] Clarke, T.R., Gibson, R.C., Barrow, G., Abel, W.D., and Barton, E.N. (2010). Depression among persons attending a HIV/AIDS outpatient clinic in Kingston, Jamaica. *West Indian Medical Journal* 59(4):369–73.

[25] Campos, L.N., Guimaraes, M.D., and Remien, R.H. (2010). Anxiety and depression symptoms as risk factors for nonadherence to antiretroviral therapy in Brazil. *AIDS and Behavior* 14(2):289–99.

[26] Khan, M.A., and Sehgal, A. (2010). Clinico-epidemiological and Socio-behavioral Study of People Living with HIV/AIDS. *Indian Journal of Psychological Medicine* 32:22-8.

[27] Sivasubramanian, M., Mimiaga, M.J., Mayer, K.H., Anand, V.R., Johnson, C.V., Prabhugate, P., and Safren, S.A. (2011). Suicidality, clinical depression, and anxiety disorders are highly prevalent in men who have sex with men in Mumbai, India: findings from a community-recruited sample. *Psychology, Health and Medicine* 16(4):450–62.

[28] Nebhinani, N., Mattoo, S.K., and Wanchu, A. (2011). Psychiatric morbidity in HIV-positive subjects: A study from India. *Journal of Psychosomatic Research* 70(5):449–54.

[29] Hasanah, C.I., Zaliha, A.R., andMahiran, M. (2011). Factors influencing the quality of life in patients with HIV in Malaysia. *Quality of Life Research: An International Journal of Quality of Life Aspects of Treatment, Care & Rehabilitation* 20(1):91–100.

[30] Morrison, S.D., Banushi, V.H., Sarnquist, C., Gashi, V.H., Osterberg, L., Maldonado, Y., andHarxhi, A. (2011). Levels of self-reported depression and anxiety among HIV-positive patients in

Albania: a cross-sectional study. *Croatian Medical Journal* 52(5):622–8.

[31] Bhatia, R., Hartman, C., Kallen, M.A., Graham, J., and Giordano, T.P. (2011). Persons newly diagnosed with HIV Infection are at high risk for depression and poor linkage to care. *AIDS and Behavior* 15(6):1161–70.

[32] Kinyanda, E., Hoskins, S., Nakku, J., Nawaz, S., and Patel, V. (2011). Prevalence and risk factors of major depressive disorder in HIV/AIDS as seen in semi-urban Entebbe district, Uganda. *BMC Psychiatry* 11:205.

[33] Agrawal, M., Srivastava, K., Goyal, S., and Chaudhury, S. (2012). Psychosocial correlates of human immunodeficiency virus infected patients. *Industrial Psychiatry Journal* 21(1):55–60.

[34] Pappin, M., Wouters, E., andBooysen, F.L. (2012). Anxiety and depression amongst patients enrolled in a public sector antiretroviral treatment programme in South Africa: a cross-sectional study. *BMC Public Health* 12:244.

[35] L'akoa, R.M., Noubiap, J.J., Fang, Y., Ntone, F.E., and Kuaban, C. (2013). Prevalence and correlates of depressive symptoms in HIV-positive patients: a cross-sectional study among newly diagnosed patients in Yaoundé, Cameroon. *BMC Psychiatry*13:228.

[36] Su, X., Lau, J.T., Mak, W.W., Choi, K.C., Chen, L., Song, J., Zhang, Y., Zhao, G., Feng, T., Chen, X., Liu, C., Liu, J., Liu, D., and Cheng, J.(2013). Prevalence and associated factors of depression among people living with HIV in two cities in China. *Journal of Affective Disorder* 149:108–15.

[37] Talukdar, A., Ghosal, M.K., Sanyal, D., Talukdar, P.S., Guha, P., Guha, S.K., and Basu, S. (2013). Determinants of quality of life in HIV-infected patients receiving highly active antiretroviral treatment at a medical college ART center in Kolkata, India. *Journal of the International Association of the Providers of AIDS Care*12(4):284–90.

[38] Olagunju, A.T., Ogundipe, O.A., Erinfolami, A.R., Akinbode, A.A., and Adeyemi, J.D. (2013). Toward the integration of comprehensive

mental health services in HIV care: an assessment of psychiatric morbidity among HIV-positive individuals in sub-Saharan Africa. *AIDS Care* 25(9):1193–8.

[39] Song, J. Y., Lee, J. S., Seo, Y. B., Kim, I. S., Noh, J. Y., Baek, J. H., Cheong, H. J., and Kim, W. J. (2013). Depression among HIV-infected patients in Korea: assessment of clinical significance and risk factors. *Infection and Chemotherapy* 45(2):211–6.

[40] Liu, L., Pang, R., Sun, W., Wu, M., Qu, P., Lu, C., and Wang, L. (2013). Functional social support, psychological capital, and depressive and anxiety symptoms among people living with HIV/AIDS employed full-time. *BMC Psychiatry* 13:324.

[41] Chauhan, V.S., Chaudhury, S., Sudarsanan, S., and Srivastava, K. (2013). Psychiatric morbidity in asymptomatic human immunodeficiency virus patients. *Industrial Psychiatry Journal* 22(2):125–30.

[42] Levy, I., Goldstein, A., Fischel, T., Maor, Y., Litachevsky, V., and Rahav, G. (2013). Neurocognitive disturbances and psychiatric disorders among patients living with HIV-1 positive in Israel. *Harefuah* 152(4):196–9.

[43] Nel, A., and Kagee, A. (2013). The relationship between depression, anxiety and medication adherence among patients receiving antiretroviral treatment in South Africa. *AIDS Care* 25(8):948–55.

[44] Largu, M.A., Dorob, C.M., Prisacariu, L., Nicolau, C., Astrstoae, V., and Manciuc, C. (2014). *The psycho-emotional profile of the HIV-positive naïve patient.* Revista medico-chirugicala a Societatii de Medici siNaturalisti din Iasi118(3):733–7.

[45] Kim, M.H., Mazenga, A.C., Devandra, A., Ahmed, S., Kazembe, P.N., Yu, X., Nguyen, C., and Sharp, C. (2014). Prevalence of depression and validation of the Beck Depression Inventory-II and the Children's Depression Inventory-Short amongst HIV-positive adolescents in Malawi. *Journal of International AIDS Society* 7:18965.

[46] Kittner, J. M., Brokamp, F, Thomaidis, T, Schmidt, R.E., Wiltink, J., Galle, P.R. and Jäger, B. (2014). Disclosure and experienced social

support are not related to anxiety or depression in a German HIV patient cohort. *Infection and Chemotherapy* 46(2):77–83.

[47] Bhatia, M.S., and Munjal, S. (2014). Prevalence of depression in people living with HIV/AIDS undergoing ART and factors associated with it. *Journal of Clinical and Diagnostic Research* 8(10):1–4.

[48] Sun, W., Wu, M., Qu, P., Lu, C., and Wang, L. (2014). Psychological well-being of people living with HIV/AIDS under the new epidemic characteristics in China and the risk factors: a population-based study. *International Journal of Infectious Disease* 28:147–52.

[49] Qiu, Y., Luo, D., Cheng, R., Xiao, Y., Chen, X., Huang, Z., and Xiao, S. (2014). *Emotional problems and related factors in patients with HIV/AIDS.* Zhong Nan Da XueXue Bao Yi Xue Ban 39(8):835–41.

[50] Glémaud, M., Illa, L., Echenique, M., Bustamente-Avellaneda, V., Gazabon, S., Villar-Loubet, O., Rodriguez, A., Potter, J., Messick, B., Jayaweera, D.T., Boulanger, C., and Kolber, M.A. (2014). Abuse and mental health concerns among HIV-infected Haitian women living in the United States. *Journal of the Association of Nurses in AIDS Care* 25(1 suppl): S62–S69.

[51] Lowther, K., Selman, L., Harding, R., Higginson, I.J. (2014). Experience of persistent psychological symptoms and perceived stigma among people with HIV on antiretroviral therapy (ART): a systematic review. *International Journal of Nursing Studies* 51(8):1171–89.

[52] Arseniou, S. Arvaniti, A., and Samakouri, M. (2014). HIV infection and depression. *Psychiatry and Clinical Neurosciences* 68: 96-109.

[53] Kosiba, J.D., Gonzalez, A., O'Cleirigh, C., and Safren, S.A. (2014). Medication adherence and HIV symptom distress in relation to panic disorder among HIV-positive adults managing opioid dependence. *Cognitive Therapy and Research* 38(4):458–64.

[54] Kee, M.K., Lee, S.Y., Kim, N.Y., Lee, J.S., Kim, J.M., Choi, J.Y., Ku, N.S., Kang, M.W., Kim, M.J., Woo, J.H., Kim, S.W., Song,

J.Y., Baek, J.H., Choi, B.Y., and Kim, S.S. (2015). Anxiety and depressive symptoms among patients infected with human immunodeficiency virus in South Korea. *AIDS Care* 27(9):1174–82.

[55] Nomoto, S. H., Longhi, R.M., de Barros, B.P., Croda, J., Ziff, E.B., Castelon, K.E. (2015). Socioeconomic disadvantage increasing risk for depression among recently diagnosed HIV patients in an urban area in Brazil: cross-sectional study. *AIDS Care* 5:1–7.

[56] Slot, M., Sodemann, M., Gabel, C., Holmskov, J., Laursen, T., and Rodkjaer, L. (2015) Factors associated with risk of depression and relevant predictors of screening for depression in clinical practice: a cross-sectional study among HIV-infected individuals in Denmark. *HIV Medicine* 16(7):393–402.

[57] Eshetu, D.A., Woldeyohannes, S.M., Kebede, M.A., Techane, G.N., Gizachew, K.D., Tegegne, M.T., and Misganaw, B.T. (2015). Prevalence of Depression and associated factors among HIV/ AIDS patients attending ART clinic at Debrebirhan Referral Hospital, North Showa, Amhara Region, Ethiopia. *Clinical Psychiatry* 1(1): 1-7.

[58] Onyebueke, G.C., and Okwaraji, F. (2015), Depression and Suicide Risk among HIV Positive Individuals Attending an Out Patient HIV/ Aids Clinic of a Nigerian Tertiary Health Institution. *Journal of Psychiatry* 18: 182.

[59] O'Cleirigh, C., Magidson, J.F., Skeer, M. R., Mayer, K. H., and Safren, S. A. (2015). Prevalence of psychiatric and substance abuse symptomatology among HIV-infected gay and bisexual men in HIV primary care. *Psychosomatics* 56(5):470-8.

[60] Ghose, T., Chowdhury, A., Solomon, P., and Ali, S. (2015). Depression and anxiety among HIV-positive sex workers in Kolkata, India: Testing and modifying the Hospital Anxiety Depression Scale. *International Social Work* 58(2): 211 –22.

[61] Tesfaw, G., Ayano, G., Awoke, T., Assefa, D., Birhanu, Z., Miheretie, G., and Abebe, G. (2016). Prevalence and correlates of depression and anxiety among patients with HIV onfollow up at Alert Hospital, Addis Ababa, Ethiopia. *BMC Psychiatry* 16:368.

[62] Radzniwan, R., Alyani, M., Aida, J., Khairani, O., Jaafar, N.R.N., and Tohid, H. (2016). Psychological status and its clinical determinants among people living with HIV/AIDS (PLWHA) in Northern Peninsular Malaysia. *HIV & AIDS Review* 15 (4): 141-6.

[63] Choi, S.K.Y., Boyle, E., Cairney, J., Collins, E.J., Gardner, S., Bacon, J., and Rourke, S.B. (2016). Prevalence, Recurrence, and Incidence of Current Depressive Symptoms among People Living with HIV in Ontario, Canada: Results from the Ontario HIV Treatment Network Cohort Study. *PLoS ONE* 11 (11): e0165816.

[64] Smith Fawzi, M.C., Ng, L., Kanyanganzi, F., Kirk, C., Bizimana, J., Cyamatare, F., Mushashi, C., Kim, T., Kayiteshonga, Y., Binagwaho, A., and Betancourt, T.S. (2016). Mental Health and Antiretroviral Adherence among Youth Living With HIV in Rwanda. *Pediatrics* 138(4):e20153235.

[65] Niu, L., Luo, D., Liu, Y., Silenzio, V.M.B., and Xiao, S. (2016). The Mental Health of People Living with HIV in China, 1998–2014: A Systematic Review. *PLoS ONE* 11(4): e0153489.

[66] Wani, M.A., and Sankar, R. (2017). Stress, anxiety and depression in HIV/AIDS patients. *Journal of Indian Health Psychology* 12 (1): 87-97.

[67] Algoodkar, S., Kidangazhiathmana, A., Rejani, P.P., and Shaji, K. S. (2017). Prevalence and factors associated with depression among clinically stable people living with HIV/AIDS on antiretroviral therapy. *Indian Journal of Psychological Medicine* 39:789-93.

[68] Kanmogne, G.D., Qiu, F., Ntone, F.E., Fonsah, J.Y., Njamnshi, D.M., Kuate, C.T., Doh, R.F., Kengne, A.M., Tagny, C.T., Nchindap, E., Kenmogne, L., Mbanya, D., Cherner, M., Heaton, R.K., and Njamnshi, A.K.(2017) Depressive symptoms in HIV-infected and seronegative control subjects in Cameroon: Effect of age, education and gender. *PLoS ONE* 12(2): e0171956.

[69] Elbadawi, A., and Mirghani, H.(2017). Depression among HIV/AIDS Sudanese patients: a cross-sectional analytic study. *The Pan African Medical Journal* 2017;26:43.

[70] Betancur, M.N., Lins, L., Oliveira, I.R., and Brites, C. (2017). Quality of life, anxiety and depression in patients with HIV/AIDS who present poor adherence to antiretroviral therapy: a cross-sectional study in Salvador, Brazil. *Brazilian Journal of Infectious Diseases* 21(5):507-14.

[71] Deshmukh, N.N., Borkar, A.M., and Deshmukh, J.S. (2017). Depression and its associated factors among people living with HIV/AIDS: Can it affect their quality of life? *Journal of Family Medicine and Primary Care* 6(3): 549–53.

[72] Egbe, C.O., Dakum, P.S., Ekong, E., Kohrt, B.A., Minto, J.G., Ticao, C.J. (2017). Depression, suicidality, and alcohol use disorder among people living with HIV/ AIDS in Nigeria. *BMC Public Health* 17:542.

[73] Tao, J., Vermund, S.H., Lu, H., Ruan, Y., Shepherd, B.E., Kipp, A.M., Amico, K.R., Zhang, X., Shao, Y., and Qian, H.Z. (2017). Impact of Depression and Anxiety on Initiation of Antiretroviral Therapy Among Men Who Have Sex with Men with Newly Diagnosed HIV Infections in China. *AIDS Patient Care and STDs* 31(2), 96-104.

[74] Kwakye, A. (2018). Prevalence and Impact of Depression, Anxiety and Stress on CD4+ Cell Counts of HIV/AIDS Patients Receiving HAART in Ghana. *Journal of AIDS and Clinical Research* 9: 781.

[75] Terloyeva, D., Nugmanova, Z., Akhmetova, G., Akanov, A., Patel, N., Lazariu, V., Norelli, L., and McNutt, L.A. (2018). Untreated depression among persons living with human immunodeficiency virus in Kazakhstan: A cross-sectional study. *PLoS ONE* 13(3): e0193976.

[76] Rane, M.S., Hong, T., Govere, S., Thulare, H., Moosa, M. Y., Celum, C., and Drain, P.K. (2018). Depression and Anxiety as Risk Factors for Delayed Care-Seeking Behavior in Human Immunodeficiency Virus–Infected Individuals in South Africa. *Clinical Infectious Diseases* 67: 1411-8.

[77] Hafeez, T. (2018). A comparative study of depression and anxiety in HIV/AIDS patients registered at treatment center in Lahore

Pakistan. *Journal of Medical Research and Biological Studies* 1: 1-6.

[78] Zhou, E., Qiao, Z., Cheng, Y., Zhou, J., Wang, W., Zhao, M., Qiu, X., Wang, L., Song, X., Zhao, E., Wang, R., Zhao, X., Yang, Y., and Yang, X. (2019). Factors associated with depression among HIV/AIDS children in China. *International Journal of Mental Health Systems* 13:10.

[79] Adeoti, A.O., Dada, M.U., and Fadare, J.O. (2018). Prevalence of Depression and Anxiety Disorders in People Living with HIV/AIDS in a Tertiary Hospital in South Western Nigeria. *Medical Reports and Case Studies* 3: 150.

[80] Wondatir, B.C., and Abdelmenan, S. (2018). Prevalence and associated factors of depression among HIV positive clients at Yekatit 12 Hospital Medical College, Addis Ababa, Ethiopia. *International Journal of Advances in Science Engineering and Technology* 6(2):38-45.

[81] Tymchuk, S., Gomez, D., Koenig, N., Gill, M.J., Fujiwara, E., and Power, C. (2018). Associations between depressive symptomatology and Neurocognitive Impairment in HIV/AIDS. *The Canadian Journal of Psychiatry* 63(5), 329-36.

[82] Kavya, R., and Badiger, S. (2018). Depression and anxiety among people living with HIV in a coastal city of Karnataka. *International Journal of Community Medicine and Public Health* 5:2931-4.

[83] Liu, H., Zhao, M., Ren, J., Qi, X., Sun, H., Qu, L., Yan, C., Zheng, T., Wu, Q., and Cui, Y. (2018).Identifying factors associated with depression among men living with HIV/ AIDS and undergoing antiretroviral therapy: a cross-sectional study in Heilongjiang, China. *Health and Quality of Life Outcomes* 16:190.

[84] Wang, T., Fu, H., Kaminga, A.C., Li, Z., Guo, G., Chen, L., and Li, Q. (2018). Prevalence of depression or depressive symptoms among people living with HIV/AIDS in China: a systematic review and meta-analysis. *BMC Psychiatry* 18:160.

[85] Ngocho, J.S., Watt, M.H., Minja, L., Knettel, B.A., Mmbaga, B.T., Williams, P.P. (2019) Depression and anxiety among pregnant

women living with HIV in Kilimanjaro region, Tanzania. *PLoS ONE* 14 (10): e0224515.

[86] Niu, L., Luo, D., Chen, X., Wang, M., Zhou, W., Zhang, D., and Xiao, S. (2019). Longitudinal trajectories of emotional problems and unmet mental health needs among people newly diagnosed with HIV in China.*Journal of the International AIDS Society* 22:e25332.

[87] Duko, B., Toma, A., Asnake, S., and Abraham, Y. (2019). Depression, Anxiety and Their Correlates among Patients with HIV in South Ethiopia: An Institution Based Cross-Sectional Study. *Frontiers Psychiatry* 10:290.

[88] Harrington, B.J., Pence, B.W., John, M., Melhado, C.G., Phulusa, J., Mthiko, B., Gaynes, B.N., Maselko, J., Miller, W.C. and Hosseinipour, M.C. (2019). Prevalence and factors associated with antenatal depressive symptoms among women enrolled in Option B+ antenatal HIV care in Malawi: a cross-sectional analysis. *Journal of Mental Health* 28(2): 198-205.

[89] Gebrezgiabher, B.B., Abraha, T.H., Hailu, E., Siyum, H., Mebrahtu, G., Gidey, B., Abay, M., Hintsa, S., and Angesom, T. (2019). Depression among Adult HIV/AIDS Patients Attending ART Clinics at Aksum Town, Aksum, Ethiopia: A Cross-Sectional Study. *Depression Research and Treatment* 2019, 3250431, 8 pages. https://doi.org/10.1155/2019/3250431.

[90] Abebe, H., Shumet, S., Nassir, Z., Agidew, M., and Abebaw, D. Prevalence of Depressive Symptoms and Associated Factors among HIV-Positive Youth Attending ART Follow-Up in Addis Ababa, Ethiopia. *AIDS Research and Treatment* 2019: 4610458, 7 pages https://doi.org/10.1155/2019/4610458.

[91] Camara, A., Sow, M.S., Touré, A., Sako, F.B., Camara, I., Soumaoro, K., Delamou, A., and Doukouré, M. (2020). Anxiety and depression among HIV patients of the infectious disease department of Conakry University Hospital in 2018. *Epidemiology and Infection* 148, e8, 1–6.

[92] Olagunju, A.T., Adeyemi, J.D., Ogbolu, R.E., and Campbell, E.A. (2012). A study on epidemiological profile of anxiety disorders

among people living with HIV/AIDS in a sub-Saharan Africa HIV clinic. *AIDS and Behaviour* 16(8):2192–2197.

[93] Ivanova, E.L., Hart, T.A., Wagner, A.C., Aljassem, K., and Loutfy, M.R. (2012). Correlates of anxiety in women living with HIV of reproductive age. *AIDS and Behavior* 16(8):2181–2191.

[94] Nurutdinova, D., Chrusciel, T., Zeringue, A., Scherrer, J.F., Al-Aly, Z., McDonald, J.R., and Overton, E.T. (2012). Mental health disorders and the risk of AIDS-defining illness and death in HIV-infected veterans. *AIDS* 26(2):229–234.

[95] Reif, S.S., Pence, B.W., LeGrand, S., Wilson, E.S., Swartz, M., Ellington, T., and Whetten, K. (2012). In-home mental health treatment for individuals with HIV. *AIDS Patient Care and STDs* 26(11):655–661.

[96] Lopes, M., Olfson, M., Rabkin, J., Hasin, D.S., Alegría, A.A., Lin, K., and Blanco, C. (2012). Gender, HIV status, and psychiatric disorders: Results from the National Epidemiologic Survey on Alcohol and Related Conditions. *Journal of Clinical Psychiatry* 73(3):384–391.

[97] Celesia, B. M., Nigro, L., Pinzone, M. R., Coco, C., La Rosa, R., Bisicchia, F., Mavilla, S., Gussio, M., Pellicanò, G., Milioni, V., Palermo, F., Russo, R., Mughini, M.T., Martellotta, F., Taibi, R., Cacopardo, B., and Nunnari, G. (2013). High prevalence of undiagnosed anxiety symptoms among HIV-positive individuals on cART: a cross-sectional study. *Eur Rev Med Pharmacol Sci* 17(15):2040–2046.

[98] Parhami, I., Fong, T.W., Siani, A., Carlotti, C., and Khanlou, H. (2013). Documentation of psychiatric disorders and related factors in a large sample population of HIV-positive patients in California. *AIDS and Behavior* 17(8):2792–801.

[99] Breuer, E., Stoloff, K., Myer, L., Seedat, S., Stein, D.J., and Joska, J.A. (2014). The validity of the Substance Abuse and Mental Illness Symptom Screener (SAMISS) in people living with HIV/AIDS in primary HIV care in Cape Town, South Africa. *AIDS and Behavior* 18(6):1133–1141.

[100] Shukla, M., Agarwal, M., Singh, J.V., and Srivastava, A.K. (2016). Anxiety among people living with HIV/AIDS on antiretroviral treatment attending tertiary care hospitals in Lucknow, Uttar Pradesh, India. *International Journal of Research in Medical Science* 4(7):2897-2901.

[101] Zisook, S., Peterkin, J., Goggin, K.J., Sledge, P., Atkinson, J.H., and Grant, I. (1998). Treatment of major depression in HIV-seropositive men. HIV Neurobehavioral Research Center Group. *Journal of Clinical Psychiatry* 59:217–24.

[102] Asch, S.M., Kilbourne, A.M., Gifford A. L., Burnam, M.A., Turner, B., Shapiro, M.F., Bozzette, S.A., and HCSUS Consortium. (2003). Under diagnosis of depression in HIV. *Journal of General Internal Medicine* 18:450–60.

[103] Burack, J.H., Barrett, D.C., Stall, R.D., Chesney, M.A., Ekstrand, M.L., and Coates, T.J. (1993). Depressive symptoms and CD4 lymphocyte decline among HIV-infected men. *JAMA* 270:2568–73.

[104] Ickovics, J.R., Hamburger, M.E., Vlahov, D., Schoenbaum, E.E., Schuman, P., Boland, R.J., Moore, J. and HIV Epidemiology Research Study Group. (2001). Mortality, CD4 cell count decline and depressive symptoms among HIV-seropositive women: longitudinal analysis from the HIV Epidemiology Research Study. *JAMA* 285:1466–74.

[105] Habib, S.E. (2004). AIDS, Sex Work and Gender: Researching Female Sex Workers in Bangladesh. In: Hossain K. T., Imam M. H., Habib S. E., editors. *Women Gender and Discrimination.* 155–170. Rajshahi: Higher Education Link Programme.

[106] Valverdee, E.E., Purcell, D., Waldrop-Valverfe, D., Knowlton, A.R., Gómez, C.A., Farrell, N., Latka, M.H., and INSPIRE Study Team. (2007). Correlates of depression among HIV-positive women and men who inject drugs. *Journal of Acquired Immune Deficiency Syndrome* 46(suppl 2):S96–S100.

[107] Frank, E, Carpenter, L.L., and Kupfer, D.J. (1998). Sex differences in recurrent depression: are there any that are significant? *American Journal of Psychiatry* 145:41–45.

[108] Young, E.A. (1990). Glucocorticoid cascade hypothesis revisited: role of gonadal steroids. *Depression* 3:20–7.

[109] Silverstein, B. (1999). Gender difference in the prevalence of clinical depression: the role played by depression associated with somatic symptoms. *American Journal of Psychiatry* 156:480–2.

[110] Ofovwe, C.E., and Ofovwe, C. (2013). Psychological disorders among human immunodeficiency virus-infected adults in southern Nigeria. *African Journal of Reproductive Health* 17(4 Spec No):177–82.

[111] Saadat, M., Behboodi, Z.M., and Saadat, E. (2015). Comparison of depression, anxiety, stress, and related factors among women and men with human immunodeficiency virus infection. *Journal of Human Reproductive Science* 8(1):48–51.

[112] Jallow, A., Ljunggren, G., Wändell, P., Carlsson, A.C. (2015). Prevalence, incidence, mortality and co-morbidities amongst human immunodeficiency virus (HIV) patients in Stockholm County, Sweden – the Greater Stockholm HIV Cohort Study. *AIDS Care* 27(2):142–149.

[113] Chandra, P.S., Desai, G., and Ranjan, S. (2005). HIV and psychiatric disorders. *Indian Journal of Medical Research* 121: 451-67.

[114] Bharat, S., and Aggeleton, P. (1999). Facing the challenge: Household responses to AIDS in Mumbai, India. *AIDS Care* 11: 31-44.

[115] Owe-Larsson, B., Sall, L., Salamon, E., and Allgulander, C. (2009). HIV infection and psychiatric illness. *African Journal of Psychiatry* (Johannesbg) 12:115–28.

[116] Atkinson, J.H., Heaton, R.K., Patterson, T.L. (2008). Two-year prospective study of major depressive disorder in HIV-infected men. *Journal of Affective Disorders* 108(3):225–34.

[117] Bozzette, S. A, Berry, S.H., Duan, N., Frankel, M.R., Leibowitz, A.A., and Lefkowitz, D. (1998). The Care of HIV-Infected Adults in the United States. *New England Journal of Medicine* 339:1897-904.

[118] Cook, J.A., Burke-Miller, J.K., Steigman, P.J., Schwartz, R.M., Hessol, N.A., Milam, J. (2018). Prevalence, Comorbidity, and

Correlates of Psychiatric and Substance Use Disorders and Associations with HIV Risk Behaviors in a Multisite Cohort of Women Living with HIV. *AIDS and Behavior* 22:3141-54.

[119] Schlebusch, L., and Vawda, N. (2010). HIV-infection as a self-reported risk factor for attempted suicide in South Africa. *African Journal of Psychiatry,* 13: 280-3.

[120] Sewell, M.C., Goggin, K.J., Rabkin, J.G., Ferrando, S.J., McElhiney, M.C., and Evans, S. (2000). Anxiety syndromes and symptoms among men with AIDS: a longitudinal controlled study. *Psychosomatics.* 41:294-300.

[121] Ferrando, S., Goggin, K., Sewell, M., Evans, S., Fishman, B., and Rabkin, J. (1998). Substance use disorders in gay/bisexual men with HIV and AIDS. *American Journal of Addiction* 7:51-60.

[122] Chandra, P.S., Ravi, V., and Desai, A. (1998). Anxiety and depression among HIV-infected heterosexuals- a report from India. *Journal of Psychosom Research* 45:401-9.

[123] Gonzalez, J.S., Batchelder, A.W., Psaros, C., and Safren, S.A. (2011). Depression and HIV/AIDS treatment nonadherence: a review and meta-analysis. *Journal of Acquired Immune Deficiency Syndrome* 58(2):181-7.

[124] Bing, E.G., Burnam, M.A., Longshore, D., Fleishman, J.A., Sherbourne, C.D, and London, A.S. (2001). Psychiatric disorders and drug use among human immunodeficiency virus-infected adults in the United States. *Archives of General Psychiatry* 58(8):721-8.

[125] Wight, R., LeBlanc, A., and de Vries, B. (2012). Stress and mental health among midlife and older gay-identified men. *Amrican Journal of Public Health* 102(3):503-10.

[126] Sherr, L., Lampe, F., Fisher, M., Arthur. G., Anderson, J., andZetler S. (2008). Suicidal ideation in UK HIV clinic attenders. *AIDS* 2008; 22(13):1651-1658.

[127] Orlando, M., Burnam, A., Beckman, R., Morton, S.C., London, A.S., Bing, E.G., and Fleishman, J.A. (2001). Re-estimating the prevalence of psychiatric disorders in a nationally representative sample of persons receiving care for HIV: results from the HIV Cost

and Services Utilization Study. *International Journal of Methods in Psychiatric Research* 11(2):75–82.

[128] Sherbourne, C.D., Hays, R.D., Fleishman, J.A., Vitiello, B., Magruder, K.M., Bing, E.G., McCaffrey, D., Burnam, A., Longshore, D., Eggan, F., Bozzette, S.A., and Shapiro, M.F. (2000). Impact of psychiatric conditions on health-related quality of life in persons with HIV infection. *American Journal of Psychiatry* 157:248–54.

[129] Tsao, J.C., Dobalian, A., Naliboff, B.D. (2004). Panic disorder and pain in a national sample of persons living with HIV. *Pain* 109:172–80.

[130] Summers, J., Zisook, S., Atkinson, J.H., Sciolla, A., Whitehall, W., Brown, S., Patterson, T., and Grant, I. (1995). Psychiatric morbidity associated with acquired immunodeficiency syndrome-related grief resolution. *Journal of Nervous and Mental Disease* 183:384–9.

[131] Haller, D.L., and Miles, D.R. (2003). Suicidal ideation among psychiatric patients with HIV: psychiatric morbidity and quality of life. *AIDS and Behavior* 7(2):101–108.

[132] Tucker, J.S., Burnam, M.A., Sherbourne, C.D., Kung, F.Y., and Gifford, A.L. (2003). Substance use and mental health correlates of nonadherence to antiretroviral medications in a sample of patients with human immunodeficiency virus infection. *American Journal of Medicine* 114:573–80.

[133] Wilkins, J.W., Robertson, K.R., Snyder, C.R., Robertson, W.K., van der Horst, C., and Hall, C.D. (1991). Implications of self-reported cognitive and motor dysfunctions in HIV-positive patients. *American Journal of Psychiatry* 148(5):641–643.

[134] Misdrahi, D., Vila, G., Funk-Brentano, I., Tardieu, M., Blanche, S., &Mouren-Simeoni, M. C. (2004). DSM-IV mental disorders and neurological complications in children and adolescents with human immunodeficiency virus type 1 infection (HIV-1). *European Psychiatry* 19(3), 182–4.

[135] Scharko, A. M. (2006). DSM psychiatric disorders in the context of pediatric HIV/AIDS. *AIDS Care* 18(5), 441–45.

[136] Mellins, C. A., Brackis-Cott, E., Dolezal, C., and Abrams, E. J. (2006). Psychiatric disorders in youth with perinatally acquired human immunodeficiency virus infection. *The Pediatric Infectious Disease Journal* 25(5), 432–7.

[137] Benton, T. D. (2011). Psychiatric considerations in children and adolescents with HIV/AIDS. *Pediatric Clinics of North America* 58(4), 989–1002.

[138] Murphy, D. A., Durako, S. J., Moscicki, A. B., Vermund, S. H., Ma, Y., Schwarz, D. F., and Adolescent Medicine HIV/AIDS Research Network. (2001). No change in health risk behaviors over time among HIV infected adolescents in care: Role of psychological distress. *The Journal of Adolescent Health* 29(3 Suppl), 57–63.

[139] DeLaMora, P., Aledort, N., &Stavola, J. (2006). Caring for adolescents with HIV. *Current HIV/AIDS Reports* 3(2), 74–78.

[140] De Maat, M. M. R., Ekhart, G. C., Huitema, A. D. R., Koks, C. H. W., Mulder, J. W., &Beijnen, J. H. (2003). Drug interactions between antiretroviral drugs and comedicated agents. *Clinical Pharmakokinetics* 42(3), 223–282.

[141] Murphy, D. A., Belzer, M., Durako, S. J., Sarr, M., Wilson, C. M., Muenz, L. R., et al. (2005). Longitudinal antiretroviral adherence among adolescents infected with human immunodeficiency virus. *Archives of Pediatrics & Adolescent Medicine* 159(8), 764–770.

[142] Williams, P. L., Storm, D., Montepiedra, G., Nichols, S., Kammerer, B., Sirois, P. A., Farley, J., and Malee, K. (2006). Predictors of adherence to antiretroviral medications in children and adolescents with HIV infection. *Pediatrics* 118(6), e1745–e1757.

[143] Nanni, M.G., Caruso, R., Mitchell, A.J., Meggiolaro, E., and Grassi, L. (2015). Depression in HIV infected patients: a review. *Current Psychiatry Reports* 17(1):530.

[144] Lyketsos, C.G., Hanson, A., Fishman, M., McHugh, P.R., and Treisman, G.J. (1994). Screening for psychiatric morbidity in a medical outpatient clinic for HIV infection: the need for a psychiatric presence. *International Journal of Psychiatry in Medicine* 24(2):103–13.

[145] Savetsky, J.B., Sullivan, L.M., Clarke, J., Stein, M.D., and Samet, J.H. (2001). Evolution of depressive symptoms in human immunodeficiency virus-infected patients entering primary care. *Journal of Nervous and Mental Disease* 189(2):76–83.

[146] Hinkin, C.H., Castellon, S.A., Atkinson, J.H., and Goodkin, K. Neuropsychiatric aspects of HIV infection among older adults. *Journal of Clinical Epidemiology* 54(suppl 1):S44–S52.

[147] de Ronchi D, Faranca I, Forti P, Ravaglia, G., Borderi, M., Manfredi, R., and Volterra, V. (2000). Development of acute psychotic disorders and HIV-1 infection. *Intenational Journal of Psychiatry in Medicine* 30(2):173–183.

[148] Khan, N., and Loewenson, R. (2005). *Guidelines for Reducing Stigma and Discrimination and Enhancing Care and Support for People Living with HIV and AIDS.* Harare: Training and Research Support Centre; South African Network of AIDS Service Organizations and European Commission.

[149] Li, L., Lee, S.J., Thammawijaya, P., Jiraphongsa, C., and Rotheram-Borus, M.J. (2009). Stigma, social support, and depression among people living with HIV in Thailand. *AIDS Care* 21(8):1007–13.

[150] Kamen. C., Arganbright, J., Kienitz, E., Weller, M., Khaylis, A., Shenkman, T., Smith, S., Koopman, C., and Gore-Felton, C. (2015). HIV-related stigma: implications for symptoms of anxiety and depression among Malawian women. *African Journal of AIDS Research* 14(1):67–73.

[151] Liu, Y., Gong, H., Yang, G., and Yan, J. (2014). *Perceived stigma, mental health and unsafe sexual behaviors of people living with HIV/AIDS.* Zhong Nan Da XueXue Bao Yi Xue Ban 39(7):658–63.

[152] Rao, D., Choi, S.W., Victorson, D., Bode, R., Peterman, A., Heinemann, A., and Cella, D. (2009). Measuring stigma across neurological conditions: the development of the stigma scale for chronic illness (SSCI). *Quality of Life Research* 18(5):585–95.

[153] Corrigan, P., Watson, A., and Barr, L. (2006). The self-stigma of mental illness: implications for self esteem and self efficacy. *Journal of Social and Clinical Psychology* 25(9):875–84.

[154] Hatzenbuehler, M.L., O'Cleirigh, C., Mayer, K.H., Mimiaga, M.J., and Safren, S.A. (2011). Prospective associations between HIV-related stigma, transmission risk behaviors, and adverse mental health outcomes in men who have sex with men. *Annals of Behavioural Medicine* 42(2):227–34.

[155] Shacham, E., Rosenburg, N., Önen, N.F., Donovan, M.F., and Overton, E.T. (2015). Persistent HIV-related stigma among an outpatient US clinic population. *International Journal of STD and AIDS* 26(4):243–50.

[156] Maedot, P., Haile, A., Lulseged, S., and Belachew, A. (2007). Determinants of vct uptake among pregnant women attending two ANC clinics in Addis Ababa City: unmatched case control study. *Ethiop Med J* 45(4):335–342.

[157] Abaynew, Y., Deribew, A., and Deribe, K. (2011). Factors associated with late presentation to HIV/AIDS care in South Wollo Zone Ethiopia: a case-control study. *AIDS Research and Therapy* 8:8.

[158] Assefa, Y., Van Damme, W., Mariam, D.H., and Kloos, H. (2010). Toward universal access to HIV counseling and testing and antiretroviral treatment in Ethiopia: looking beyond HIV testing and ART initiation. *AIDS Patient Care and STDS* 24(8):521–525.

[159] Biadgilign, S., Deribew, A., Amberbir, A., and Deribe, K. (2009). Barriers and facilitators to antiretroviral medication adherence among HIV-infected paediatric patients in Ethiopia: a qualitative study. *Sahara Journal* 6(4): 148–54.

[160] Busby, K.K., Lytle, S., and Sajatovic, M. (2013). Mental Health Comorbidity and HIV/AIDS. In: *Mental Health Practitioner's Guide to HIV/AIDS*. Sana Loue (editor). Pp 9-36. Springer: New York.

[161] Maes, M., Kubera, M., Obuchowiczwa, E., Goehler, L., and Brzeszcz, J. (2011). Depression's multiple comorbidities explained by (neuro) inflammatory and oxidative and nitrosative stress pathways. *Neuroendocrinology Letter* 32(1):7–24.

[162] Fauci, A. S., Mavilio, D., and Kottilil, S. (2005). NK cells in HIV infection: Paradigm for protection or targets for ambush. *Nature Reviews Immunology,* 5(11), 835–843.

[163] Benton, T., Lynch, K., Dube, B., Gettes, D. R., Tustin, N. B., Ping Lai, J., Metzger, D. S., Blume, J., Douglas, S. D., and Evans, D. L. (2010). Selective serotonin reuptake inhibitor suppression of HIV infectivity and replication. *Psychosomatic Medicine* 72(9): 925–32.

[164] DelGuerra, F.B., Fonseca, J.L., Figueiredo, V.M., Ziff, E.B., Konkiewitz, E.C. (2013). Human immunodeficiency virus-associated depression: contributions of immuno-inflammatory, monoaminergic, neuro-degenerative, and neurotrophic pathways. *Journal of Neurovirology* 19(4):314–27.

[165] Schuster, R., Bornovalova, M., and Hunt, E. (2012). The influence of depression on the progression of HIV: Direct and indirect effects. *Behavior Modification* 36(2):123–45.

[166] McGuire, J.L., Kempen, J.H., Localio, R., Ellenberg, J.H., and Douglas, S.D. (2015). Immune markers predictive of neuropsychiatric symptoms in HIV-infected youth. *Clinical and Vaccine Immunology* 22(1):27–36.

[167] Cruess, D. G., Douglas, S. D., Petitto, J. M., Have, T. T., Gettes, D., Dube, B., Carry, M., and Evans, D.L. (2005). Association of resolution of major depression with increased natural killer cell activity among HIV-seropositive women. *The American Journal of Psychiatry* 162(11), 2125–30.

[168] Wulsin, L.R., Vaillant, G.E., Wells, V.E. (1999). A systematic review of the mortality of depression. *Psychosom Medicine* 61:6–17.

[169] Katon, W.J. (2003). Clinical and health services relationships between major depression, depressive symptoms, and general medical illness. *Biological Psychiatry* 54:216–26.

[170] Treisman, G., and Angelino, A. (2007). Interrelation between psychiatric disorders and the prevention and treatment of HIV infection. *Clinical Infectious Disease* 45(suppl 4):S313–S317.

[171] Sternhell, P.S., and Corr, M.J. (2002). Psychiatric morbidity and adherence to antiretroviral medication in patients with HIV/AIDS. *Australia & New Zealand Journal of Psychiatry* 36:528–533.

[172] Adejumo, O., Oladeji, B., Akpa, O., Malee, K., Baiyewu, O., Ogunniyi, A., Evans, S., Berzins, B., and Taiwo, B. (2016). Psychiatric disorders and adherence to antiretroviral therapy among a population of HIV-infected adults in Nigeria. *International Journal of STD & AIDS* 27(11):938-49.

[173] Springer, S.A., Dushaj, A., and Azar, M.M. (2012). The impact of DSM-IV mental disorders on adherence to combination antiretroviral therapy among adult persons living with HIV/AIDS: a systematic review. *AIDS and Behavior* 16(8):2119–2143.

[174] Paterson, D.L., Swindells, S., Mohr, J., Brester, M., Vergis, E.N., Squier, C., Wagener, M.M., and Singh, N. (2000). Adherence to protease inhibitor therapy and outcomes in patients with HIV infection. *Annals of Internal Medicine* 133:21–30.

[175] Leserman, J. (2003). HIV disease progression: depression, stress, and possible mechanisms. *Biological Psychiatry* 54:295–306.

[176] Evans, D.L., TenHave, T.R., Douglas, S.D., Gettes, D.R., Morrison, M., Chiappini, M.S., Brinker-Spence, P., Job, C., Mercer, D.E., Wang, Y.L., Cruess, D., Dube, B., Dalen, E.A., Brown, T., Bauer, R., and Petitto, J.M. (2002). Association of depression with viral load, CDS T lymphocytes and natural killer cells in women with HIV infection. *American Journal of Psychiatry* 159:1752–9.

[177] Ironson, G., Balbin, E., Solomon, G., Fahey, J., Klimas, N., Schneiderman, N., and Fletcher, M.A. (2001). Relative preservation of natural killer cell cytotoxicity and number in healthy AIDS patients with low CD4 cell counts. *AIDS* 15(16):2065–73.

[178] Cruess, D.G., Douglas, S.D., Petitto, J.M., Have, T.T., Gettes, D., Dubé, B., Cary, M., and Evans, D.L. (2005). Association of resolution of major depression with increased natural killer cell activity among HIV-seropositive women. *American Journal of Psychiatry* 162(11):2125–30.

[179] Grossman, F., and Potter, W.Z. (1999). Catecholamines in depression: a cumulative study of urinary norepinephrine and its major metabolites in unipolar and bipolar depressed patients versus healthy volunteers at the NIMH. *Psychiatry Research* 87:21–7.

[180] Cook J. A., Grey D, Burke J, Cohen, M.H., Gurtman, A.C., Richardson, J.L., Wilson, T.E., Young, M.A, and Hessol, N.A. (2004). Depressive symptoms and AIDS-related mortality among a multisite cohort of HIV-positive women. *American Journal of Public Health* 94:1133–1140.

[181] Ammassari, A., Antinori, A., Aloisi, M.S., Trotta, M.P., Murri, R., Bartoli, L., Monforte, A.D., Wu, A.W., and Starace, F. (2004). Depressive symptoms, neurocognitive impairment, and adherence to highly active antiretroviral therapy among HIV-infected persons. *Psychosomatics* 45: 394–402.

[182] Starace, F., Ammassari, A., Trotta, M.P., Murri, R., De Longis, P., Izzo, C., Scalzini, A., d'Arminio Monforte, A., Wu, A.W., Antinori, A., and AdICoNA Study Group. NeuroICoNA Study Group. (2002). Depression is a risk factor for suboptimal adherence to highly active antiretroviral therapy. *Journal of Acquired Immune Deficiency Syndrome* 31(suppl 3):s136–s139.

[183] Waldrop-Valverde, D., and Valverde, E. (2005). Homelessness and psychological distress as contributors to antiretroviral nonadherence in HIV-positive injecting drug users. *AIDS Patient Care and STDs* 19:326–34.

[184] Kacanek, D., Jacobson, D.L., Spiegelman, D., Wanke, C., Isaac, R., and Wilson, I.B. (2010). Incident depression symptoms are associated with poorer HAART adherence: a longitudinal analysis from the Nutrition for Healthy Living study. *Journal of Acquired Immune Deficiency Syndrome* 53:266–72.

[185] Horberg, M.A., Silverberg, M.J., Hurley, L.B., Towner, W.J., Klein, D.B., Bersoff-Matcha, S., Weinberg, W.G., Antoniskis, D., Mogyoros, M., Dodge, W.T., Dobrinich, R., Quesenberry, C.P., and Kovach, D.A. (2008). Effects of depression and selective serotonin reuptake inhibitor use on adherence to highly active antiretroviral

therapy and on clinical outcomes in HIV-infected patients. *Journal of Acquired Immune Deficiency Syndrome* 47(3):384–90.

[186] Dalessandro, M., Conti, C. M., Gambi, F., Falasca, K., Doyle, R., Conti, P., Caciagli, F., Fulcheri, M., and Vecchiet, J. (2007). Antidepressant therapy can improve adherence to antiretroviral regimens among HIV-infected and depressed patients. *Journal of Clinical Psychopharmacology* 27(1), 58–61.

[187] Nüesch, R., Gayet-Ageron, A., Chetchotisakd, P., Prasithsirikul, W., Kiertiburanakul, S., Munsakul, W., Raksakulkarn, P., Tansuphasawasdikul, S., Chautrakarn, S., Ruxrungthan, K., Hirschel, B., and Anaworanich, I. (2009). The Impact of Combination Antiretroviral Therapy and its Interruption on Anxiety, Stress, Depression and Quality of Life in Thai Patients.*The Open AIDS Journal* 3:38-45.

[188] Mothapo, K.M., Schellekens, A., van Crevel, R., Keuter, M., Grintjes-Huisman, K., Koopmans, P., and van der Ven, A. (2015). Improvement of depression and anxiety after discontinuation of long-term efavirenz treatment. *CNS & Neurological Disorders Drug Targets* 14(6):811–8.

[189] Pedrol, E., Llibre, J.M., Tasias, M., Currán, A., Guardiola, J.M., Deig, E., Guelar, A., Martínez-Madrid, O., Tikhomirova, L., Ramírez, R., and RELAX Study Group. (2015). Outcome of neuropsychiatric symptoms related to an antiretroviral drug following its substitution by nevirapine: the RELAX study. *HIV Medicine* 16(10):628–34.

[190] Repetto, M.J., and Petitto, J.M. (2008). Psychopharmacology in HIV-infected patients. *Psychosomatic Medicine* 70(5):585–92.

[191] Gallego, L., Barreiro, P., Lopez-Ibor, J.J. (2012). Psychopharmacological treatments in HIV patients under antiretroviral therapy. *AIDS Review* 14:101–11.

[192] Kang, E., Delzell, D.A., Chhabra, M., and Oberdorfer, P. (2015). Factors associated with high rates of antiretroviral medication adherence among youth living with perinatal HIV in Thailand. *International Journal of STD & AIDS* 26(8):534–41.

[193] Olatunji, B. O., Mimiaga, M. J., O'Cleirigh, C., &Safren, S. A. (2006). Review of treatment studies of depression in HIV. *Topics in HIV Medicine* 14(3), 112–24.

[194] Psaros, C., Israel, J., O'Cleirigh, C., Bedoya, C. A., &Safren, S. A. (2011). Psychological co-morbidities of HIV/AIDS. In S. Pagoto (Ed.), *Psychological co-morbidities of physical illness: A behavioral medicine perspective* (pp. 233–273). New York, NY: Springer Science + Business Media LLC.

[195] Repetto, M. J., and Petitto, J. M. (2008). Psychopharmacology in HIV-infected patients. *Psychosomatic Medicine* 70(5), 585–92.

[196] Mainie, I., McGurk, C., McClintock, G., & Robinson, J. (2001). Seizures after buproprion overdose. *Lancet* 357(9268), 1624.

[197] Yanofski, J., &Croarkin, P. (2008). Choosing antidepressants for HIV and AIDS patients: Insights on safety and side effects. *Psychiatry* (Edgmont (PA: Township)), 5(5), 61–66.

[198] Ferrando, S. J. (2005). Managing depression in HIV disease, viral hepatitis, and substance abuse. *The PRN Notebook* 10(4). Retrieved Jan 2, 2020 fromhttp://www.prn.org/images/pdfs/70_663_ferrando_stephen_v10_n4.pdf.

[199] Department of Health and Human Services. (2017). *Guidelines for the Use of Antiretroviral Agents in Adults and Adolescents Living with HIV.* 1-32. http://wwwaidsinfonihgov/ContentFiles/AdultandAdolescentGLpdf.

[200] Freudenreich, O., Goforth, H., Cozza, K., Mimiaga, M. J., Safren, S.A., Bachmann, G., and Cohen, M.A. (2010). Psychiatric treatment of persons with HIV/AIDS: an HIV-psychiatry consensus survey of current practices. *Psychosomatics* 51:480–488.

[201] Omonuwa, T., Goforth, H., Preud'homme, X., and Krystal, A.D. (2009). The pharmacological management of insomnia in patients with HIV. *Journal of Clinical Sleep Medicine* 5:251–62.

[202] Batki, S. (1990). Buspirone in drug users with AIDS or AIDS – related complex. *Journal of Clinical Psychopharmacology* 10:111–5.

[203] Greenblatt, D., von Moltke, L., Harmatz J., Durol, A.L., Daily, J.P., Graf, J.A., Mertzanis, P., Hoffman, J.L., and Shader, R.I. (2000). Differential impairment of triazolam and zolpidem clearance by ritonavir. *Journal of Acquired Immune Deficiency Syndrome* 24:129–36.

[204] Anderson, I. (2000). Selective serotonin reuptake inhibitors versus tricyclic antidepressants; a meta-analysis of efficacy and tolerability. *Journal of Affective Disorder* 58:19–36.

[205] Isacsson, G., Holmgren, P., and Ahlner, J. (2005). Selective serotonin reuptake inhibitor antidepressants and the risk of suicide: a controlled forensic database study of 14,857 suicides. *Acta Psychiatrica Scandanavica* 111: 286–90.

[206] Currier, M., Molina, G., and Kato, M. (2004). Citalopram treatment of major depressive disorder in Hispanic HIV and AIDS patients: a prospective study. *Psychosomatics* 45:210–6.

[207] Grassi, B., Gambini, O., Garghentini, G., Lazzarin, A., and Scarone, S. (1997). Efficacy of paroxetine for treatment of depression in the context of HIV infection. *Pharmacotherapy* 30:70–1.

[208] Fernando, S., Rabkin, J., de Moore, G., and Rabkin, R. (1999). Antidepressant treatment of depression in HIV seropositive women. *Journal of Clinical Psychiatry* 60:741–46.

[209] Baker, G., Fang, H., Sinha, S., and Coults, R. (1998). Metabolic drug interactions with selective serotonin reuptake inhibitor (SSRI) antidepressants. *Neuroscience Biobehavior Review* 22:325–33.

[210] Caballero, J., and Nahata, M. (2005). Use of selective serotonin-reuptake inhibitors in the treatment of depression in adults with HIV. *Annals of Pharmacotherapy* 39:141–145.

[211] DeSilva, K.E., Le Flore, D.B., Marston, B.J., and Rimland, D. (2001). Serotonin syndrome in HIV-infected individuals receiving antiretroviral therapy and fluoxetine. *AIDS* 15:1281–5.

[212] Elliott, A.J., Russo, J., Bergam, K., Claypoole, K., Uldall, K.K., and Roy-Byrne, P.P. (1999). Antidepressant efficacy in HIV seropositive outpatients with major depressive disorder: an open trial of nefazodone. *Journal of Clinical Psychiatry* 60(4):226–31.

[213] Currier, M., Molina, G., and Kato, M. (2003). A prospective trial of sustained release bupropion for depression in HIV-seropositive and AIDS patients. *Psychosomatics* 44:120–5.

[214] Hesse, L.M., von Moltke, L.L., Shader, R.I., and Greenblatt, D.J. (2001). Ritonavir, efavirenz, and nelfinavir inhibit CYP2B6 activity in vitro: potential drug interactions with bupropion. *Drug Metabolism & Disposal* 29:100–2.

[215] Fernandez, F., Levy, J.K., Samley, H.R., Pirozzolo, F.J., Lachar, D., Crowley, J., Adams, S., Ross, B., and Ruiz, P. (1995). Effects of methylphenidate in HIV-related depression: a comparative trial with desipramine. *International Journal of Psychiatry in Medicine* 25:53–67.

[216] Wagner, G.J., and Rabkin, R. (2000). Effects of dextroamphetamine on depression and fatigue in men with HIV: a double-blind, placebo-controlled trial. *Journal of Clinical Psychiatry* 61:436–40.

[217] Rabkin, J.G., Ferrando, S.J., Wagner, G.J., and Rabkin, R. (2000). DHEA treatment for HIV patients: effects on mood, androgenic and anabolic parameters. *Psychoneuroendocrinology* 25:53–68.

[218] Lee, M.R., Cohen, L., Hadley, S.W., and Goodwin, F.K. (1999). Cognitive-behavioral group therapy with medication for depressed gay men with AIDS or symptomatic HIV infection. *Psychiatric Services* 50:948–52.

[219] Crepaz, N., Passin W. F., Herbst J. H., Rama, S.M., Malow, R.M., Purcell, D.W., Wolitski, R.J. and HIV/AIDS Prevention Research Synthesis Team. (2008) Meta-analysis of cognitive-behavioral interventions on HIV-positive persons' mental health and immune functioning. *Health Psychology* 27(1):4–14.

[220] Spies, G., Asmal, L., and Seedat, S. (2013). Cognitive-behavioural interventions for mood and anxiety disorders in HIV: a systematic review. *Journal of Affective Disorder* 150(2):171–80.

[221] Markowitz, J.C., Klerman, G.L., Clougherty, K.F., Spielman, L.A., Jacobsberg, L.B., Fishman, B., Frances, A.J., Kocsis, J.H., and Perry, S.W. (1995).Individual psychotherapies for depressed HIV positive patients. *American Journal of Psychiatry* 152:1504–9.

[222] Markowitz, J.C., Kocsis, J.H., Fishman, B., Spielman, L.A., Jacobsberg, L.B., Frances, A.J., Klerman, G.L., and Perry, S.W. (1998). Treatment of depressive symptoms in human immunodeficiency virus-positive patient. *Archives of General Psychiatry* 55:452–7.

[223] Rousaud, A., Blanch, J., Hautzinger, M., De Lazzari, E., Peri, J.M., Puig, O., Martinez, E., Masana, G., De Pablo, J., and Gatell, J.M. (2007). Improvement of psychosocial adjustment to HIV-1 infection through a cognitive-behavioral oriented group psychotherapy program: a pilot study. *AIDS Patient Care and STDs* 21(3):212–22.

[224] Mulder, C.L., Emmelkamp, P.M., Antoni, M.H., Mulder, J.W., Sandfort, T.G,, and de Vries, M.J. (1994). Cognitive behavioral and experiential group psychotherapy for HIV-infected homosexual men: a comparative study. *Psychosomatic Medicine* 56:423–31.

[225] Honagodu, A.R., Krishna, M., Sundarachar, R., and Lepping, P. (2013). Group psychotherapies for depression in persons with HIV: A systematic review. *Indian Journal of Psychiatry* 55(4): 323–30.

[226] Brown, J.L., and Vanable, P.A. (2008). Cognitive-behavioral stress management interventions for persons living with HIV: a review and critique of the literature. *Annals of Behavioral Medicine* 35(1):26–40.

[227] Berger, S., Schad, T., von Wyl, V., Ehlert, U., Zellweger, C., Furrer, H., Regli, D., Vernazza, P., Ledergerber, B., Battegay, M., Weber, R., and Gaab, J. (2008). Effects of cognitive behavioral stress management on HIV-1 RNA, CD4 cell counts and psychosocial parameters of HIV-infected persons. *AIDS* 22(6):767–75.

[228] Vance, D.E., Humphrey, S.C., Nicholson, W. C., and Jablonski-Jaudon, R. (2014). Can speed of processing training ameliorate depressive symptomatology in adults with HIV? *Annals of Depression and Anxiety* 1(3):4.

[229] Scott-Sheldon, L.A., Kalichman, S.C., Carey, M.P., and Fielder, R.L. (2008). Stress management interventions for HIV+ adults: a meta-analysis of randomized controlled trials, 1989 to 2006. *Health Psychology* 27(2):129–139.

[230] HemmatiSabet, A., Khalatbari, J., Abbas Ghorbani, M., Haghighi, M., and Ahmadpanah, M. (2013). Group training of stress management vs. group cognitive-behavioral therapy in reducing depression, anxiety and perceived stress among HIV-positive men. *Iranian Journal of Psychiatry & Behavioral Science* 7(1):4–8.

[231] Scott-Sheldona, L.A.J., Ballettoa, B.L., Donahuea, M.L., Feulnera, M.M., Cruessd, D.G., Salmoirago-Blotchera, E., Wing, R.R., and Careya, M.P. (2019). Mindfulness-Based Interventions for Adults Living with HIV/AIDS: A Systematic Review and Meta-Analysis. *AIDS and Behavior* 23(1): 60–75.

[232] Neidig, J.L., Smith, B.A., Brashers, D.E. (2003). Aerobic exercise training for depressive symptom management in adults living with HIV infection. *Journal of Association of Nurses for AIDS Care* 14:30-40.

[233] LaPerriere, A., Klimas, N., Fletcher, M.A., Perry, A., Ironson, G., Perna, F., and Schneiderman, N. (1997). Change in CD4+ cell enumeration following aerobic exercise training in HIV-1 disease: possible mechanisms and practical applications. *International Journal of Sports Medicine* 18(suppl 1):S56-S61.

[234] LaPerriere, A., Ironson, G., Antoni, M.H., Schneiderman, N., Klimas, N., and Fletcher, M.A. (1994). Exercise and psychoneuro-immunology. *Medicine and Science in Sports and Exercise* 26:182-90.

[235] Jaggers, J.R., and Hand, G.A. (2016). Health Benefits of Exercise for People Living With HIV. A Review of the Literature. *American Journal of Lifestyle Medicine* 10(3): 184–92.

[236] Luenen, S. V., Garnefski, N., Spinhoven, P., Spaan, P., Dusseldorp, E., and Kraaij, V. (2018). The Benefits of Psychosocial Interventions for Mental Health in People Living with HIV: A Systematic Review and Meta-analysis. *AIDS and Behaviour* 22:9–42.

In: HIV/AIDS
Editor: Ethel K. Hebert

ISBN: 978-1-53617-923-1
© 2020 Nova Science Publishers, Inc.

Chapter 2

SOCIO-PSYCHOLOGICAL DETERMINANTS OF DENTAL CARE FOR PATIENTS WITH HIV

Anastasiya Sergeevna Belyakova[1,*],
Marina Vladlenovna Kozlova[1],
Igor Vladimirovich Pchelin[2]
and Kirill Aleksandrovich Barsky[2]

[1]Central State Medical Academy of the Department of Presidential Affairs, Moscow, Russia
[2]Regional Public Aid Foundation for AIDS, "Steps," Moscow, Russia

ABSTRACT

The article presents an analysis of the data of sociological research, the purpose of which was to show the prevalence of stigma and discrimination against patients with HIV infection at the dental attendance. According to the results of a voluntary face-to-face individual anonymous survey of 1268 people, living with HIV, aged 18 years and older, there was a high level (66.7%) of stigma and discrimination in medical organizations providing dental care. Fear of stigma has been a

---

[*] Corresponding Author's Email: bel.stom@mail.ru.

key factor in reducing the willingness to disclose HIV status. 36.5% of respondents do not believe in the principle of confidentiality, they are out of concern for the disclosure of the diagnosis and the consequences associated with it. In this regard, only 22.4% of those interviewed for dental care reported having HIV infection. 29.9% of respondents were asked to take an HIV test - 60% of them voluntarily, 15% in an ultimatum form, 25% of patients were under pressure. A large number of acts of discrimination were revealed in the form of a negative attitude of a physician to patients with HIV infection (25% of cases) and refusal to treat oral diseases (41.7% of cases). According to the results of the survey, the doctors, having learned about the positive HIV status of the patient, refused mainly (94%) dental surgery (tooth extraction and dental implantation). There was a high proportion of people (64.2%) who postponed the visit to the dentist due to social concerns related to their HIV status. The data of the presented study actualize the necessity for development and realization of programs to eradicate stigma and discrimination towards people living with HIV in order to timely provide qualified medical dental care, improve oral health and the quality of life of these patients.

Keywords: HIV infection, people living with HIV, stigma, discrimination, dentistry

Abbreviations

HIV	human immunodeficiency virus
WHO	World Health Organization
PLHIV	people living with HIV
AIDS	Acquired Immune Deficiency Syndrome
UNAIDS	Joint United Nations Program on HIV/AIDS

Introduction

Modern global trends are focused on improving health and maintaining a high level of life quality of the population. However, people living with HIV (PLHIV) face many barriers to accessing medical services (including dental care). Despite some efforts to reduce stigma and discrimination due to HIV, these social phenomena continue to spread in relation to both the disease itself and HIV patients (Emlet 2005; Hatzenbuehler et al. 2013).

Stigma is a quality or a characteristic of an individual, which is defined by him as unacceptable, negative (Knuf, Epov 2006). UNAIDS (The Joint United Nations Programme on HIV/AIDS) characterizes stigma as a dynamic personality depreciation process that results in discrimination - any form of exclusion or restriction of a person based on his real or perceived HIV status (UNAIDS 2005). Discrimination can occur in intentional action or inaction, and is directed against those who are stigmatized. Integration of external (negative perception from the society) and internal (negative self-perception) stigma often leads to adverse mental and social consequences. Shame, inferiority, social isolation can lead to the development of depression until the occurrence of suicidal thoughts (Stutterheim et al. 2009; Mak et al. 2007; Corrigan, Watson 2002).

Studies on stigma and discrimination when seeking medical help indicate their high level (from 36 to 59.3%) in relation to PLHIV (Ruziev et al. 2018; Research Report 2010). Fear of condemnation, rejection, humiliation, refusal of treatment and/or changes in attitudes on the part of health workers, as well as concerns about confidentiality may entail concealment of the diagnosis, which makes it difficult to diagnose and treat various kinds of concomitant pathology in this population group (Gesesew et al. al. 2017; Giuliani et al. 2005). In this regard, 54-73% of PLHIV are afraid to disclose their HIV status to a doctor (Ruziev et al. 2018).

Up to 45.9% of HIV-positive cases of medical care became a serious problem (Ruziev et al. 2018). The health care worker's own infectious safety is one of the reasons for fear of treating an HIV-infected patient, discriminatory unprofessional behavior that violates human rights, which can result in reduced quality of services provided and denial of treatment (Brondani et al. 2016; Chernyavskaya, Ioannidi 2014).

Stigma and discrimination present in the medical environment, are generally recognized barriers to PLHIV access to prevention and treatment, associated with their low accessibility of the health services they need (Ioannidi et al. 2013; Pokrovsky 2013; Bogachanskaya 2011; Logie,

Gadalla 2009). According to the report on the study of the stigma index in the Russian Federation, 22% of respondents decided not to visit medical institutions, 17% postponed seeking medical help (Research Report Moscow 2010). According to the results of the meta-analysis of H. A. Gesesew PLHIV who experience a high level of stigma are 2.4 times more likely to tolerate the start of treatment until their condition becomes seriously worse (Gesesew et al. 2017).

One of the main indicators of general health, well-being and quality of life is dental health, which WHO defines as a condition characterized by the absence of chronic pain in the oral cavity and in the face, infections and oral ulcers, periodontal diseases (gums), caries, tooth loss and other diseases and disorders that limit a person's ability to chew, smile, and talk, as well as his psychosocial well-being (Bazikyan 2009; Popova et al. 2008; Kirsanova et al. 2007; World Health Organization 2003). Due to the prevalence of stigmatization and discrimination of HIV-infected people in health care organizations, there is a disparity in the level of oral health and access to dental care, which is recognized as unfair and illegal in modern society (Dougall et al. 2018; World Health Organization 2010).

M. Choromańska, D. Waszkiel noted a higher (up to 71%) percentage of missing teeth in the group of HIV-infected people in comparison with patients without immunodeficiency, the number of people using dentures was twice as high as the control group. Reconstruction of the dentition of the upper and lower jaws was necessary in 46.94% of cases (Choromańska, Waszkiel 2006). In 30-80% of PLHIV, primary manifestations of HIV infection are observed in the form of various diseases of the oral mucosa, which, due to etiology and pathogenesis (including a tendency to relapse, a high degree of malignancy), occupy an important place in the structure of dental morbidity (Gazhva et al. 2014; Reznik 2005). Timely provision of quality medical dental care to PLHIV can significantly improve oral health and the quality of life of this category of patients.

Thus, it is relevant to study the current state of the problem of stigmatization and discrimination of PLHIV when applying for dental care.

The objective of the study is to assess the prevalence of stigma and discrimination in relation to patients with HIV infection at a dental appointment.

METHODS

On the basis of the social-information center of the Regional Charitable Foundation for the Fight against AIDS "Steps," a voluntary individual anonymous questionnaire was conducted for 1268 people living with HIV aged 18 years and older who have applied for dental care in the last 12 months. The questionnaire contained questions with pre-defined answers.

Statistical analysis of the data was carried out in the software STATISTICA 6.0 (StatSoft, Ink., USA).

RESULTS

According to the obtained data, 77.6% of survey participants did not report their HIV status before dental treatment (34.6% of patients do not consider this necessary; 63.4% are afraid of poor attitude of health workers; 34.6% believe that they know the doctor that HIV infection may have a negative impact on the quality of treatment, 36.5% do not believe in the principle of confidentiality, fear of disclosure of the diagnosis and consequences associated with this).

At the same time, 66.7% of HIV-infected people noted that when they applied for dental care, if their status was disclosed, problems related to refusal of treatment (41.7%) and negative doctor attitudes (25%) arose. According to the results of the survey, the doctors, having learned about the positive HIV status of the patient, refused mainly (94%) dental surgery (tooth extraction and dental implantation).

When requesting dental care, 29.9% of respondents were asked to take an HIV test, of which 60% voluntarily, 15% in the ultimatum form, and 25% of PLHIV were under pressure.

An analysis of the structure of needs in dental care revealed that 37.3% of respondents applied for the treating teeth; 53.7% about tooth extraction; 25.4% for dental implantation; 11.9% for orthopedic treatment; 28.4% for professional hygiene.

There was a high proportion of people (64.2%) who postponed their visit to the dentist due to fears related to their HIV status (stigmatization, refusal of treatment, disclosure of diagnosis, etc.).

Conclusion

A sociological study showed that despite the commitment to protecting human rights and political initiatives aimed at eliminating stigma and discrimination at all levels and in various areas of activity, the prevalence of these sociological phenomena in the medical (dental) environment remains high today (up to 66.7%).

Fear of stigma, stigmatizing beliefs, supported by cases of negative attitudes on the part of medical personnel, adversely affect readiness to disclose HIV status. Only 22.4% of respondents reported having HIV infection when seeking dental care.

A serious problem is the increase in the number of acts of discrimination in the form of a negative attitude of the doctor (25% of cases) to patients with HIV infection and refusal to treat oral diseases (41.7% of cases) to this group of patients. Prohibiting, hindering and refusing PLHIV to access the necessary range of medical services within the competence of a doctor contradicts modern knowledge of public health and international standards that recognize equal rights to health care and medical care for all people regardless of their HIV status. 40% of respondents encountered violations of the principle of voluntary testing for HIV when applying for dental treatment.

Fears of PLHIV in connection with their status affect their unwillingness to receive the necessary dental care, which is manifested in the postponement and repeated postponement of a doctor's appointment in 64.2% of cases. Late initiation of treatment may contribute to a greater prevalence of dental pathology (including acute inflammatory processes) in HIV-infected patients as compared with patients without immunodeficiency. Thus, early detection and timely, high-quality rational medical care are an important component in maintaining dental health and a high level of quality of life for PLHIV.

A high level of fear of disclosing a diagnosis of HIV infection was noted (36.5%). Violation of the principle of confidentiality can lead to various negative consequences in all aspects of a person's life with HIV and its environment, dramatically increasing its degree of social vulnerability. Along with discrimination at the level of institutional organizations (at workplaces, in medical institutions, educational institutions and social services), a large number of cases were reported when significant psychological pressure was put on people because of their positive HIV status; the avoidance of these people by family members, peers and society as a whole; negative attitudes and degrading human actions were manifested; there were threats to health and life (United Nations Development Program (UNDP) 2008; (UNAIDS 2005). Such illegal actions can greatly increase vulnerability and exacerbate the effects of HIV infection, which, in turn, reduces the effectiveness of the response to the epidemic.

In accordance with the Russian legislation, the violation of the rights of people living with HIV, including disclosure of the diagnosis of the disease, the results of medical examinations and treatment regimens entails the administrative and other responsibility of the medical worker. However, today, along with the knowledge of the majority of PLHIV about the existence of legal documents defining the obligations of the state regarding their protection, fear of public stigma and its consequences prevails, which prevents the appeal of this category of persons to the appropriate instances of violation of their rights.

Overcoming stigma and discrimination against HIV-infected people in the health care system can be enhanced by increasing the level of knowledge of healthcare professionals on HIV/AIDS. Today, antiretroviral therapy allows for recovery of the immune status with maximum suppression of viral replication in cells of the immune system (undetectable viral load) and the absence of clinical manifestation (Pokrovsky 2013; Belyakov, Rakhmanova 2011). Successful treatment of HIV infection (reducing the level of viremia to an undetectable level) is highly effective in preventing transmission of the virus, as confirmed by randomized, multicenter studies and controlled clinical trials (Fleming et al. 2016; Safren et al. 2015).

Education, focused on developing the competence of HIV/AIDS in health care workers (training in epidemiology, prevention of modern methods of treating HIV infection, occupational risks, etc.), informing about the negative effects of discriminatory actions is an important condition for increasing the tolerance to PLHIV that It has a significant impact on the ability to provide qualified assistance to this category of patients and to improve the quality of medical services provided.

A feature of the professional activity of the dentist is direct contact with biological fluids (blood, saliva), which accompany most dental procedures, which is a risk factor for HIV transmission. Therefore, the need to increase the level of social guarantees and the provision of means to comply with universal security measures and prevent HIV infection in the workplace are of particular importance.

It should be noted that despite all the problems and obstacles, 35.8% of PLHIV continue to seek dental care, strive for optimal oral health and try to overcome the difficulties associated with their diagnosis of HIV infection.

Thus, today there is a high level of stigma and discrimination associated with the problems of HIV infection in the segment of medical organizations that provide dental care. Given the particular seriousness of the consequences of these social phenomena, it is necessary to intensify efforts to weaken the stigmatizing attitude and discriminatory behavior towards PLHIV by health professionals at the dental reception, as well as to raise awareness of modern methods of treating and preventing HIV infection, including areas of occupational hazards.

REFERENCES

Bazikyan, E. A. (ed.), Robustova, T. G., Lukina, G. I. et al. (2009) *Procedural dentistry. Textbook.* Moscow: GEOTAR-Media.

Belyakov, N. A., Rakhmanova, A. G. (Ed.) (2011) *Human Immunodeficiency Virus - Medicine: A Guide for Physicians.* St. Petersburg: Baltic Medical Education Center.

Bogachanskaya, N. N. (2011) Attitude of general practitioners to HIV-infected patients. *Modern studies of social problems*, 1(05): 217-219.

Brondani, M. A., Phillips, J. C., Kerston, R. P., Moniri, N. R. (2016) Stigma around hiv in dental care: patients' experiences. *J. Can. Dent. Assoc.*, 82:g1.

Chernyavskaya, O. A., Ioannidi, E. A. (2014) Some aspects of stigma and discrimination of people living with HIV/AIDS. *Sociology of Medicine*, 13(2): 46-48.

Choromańska, M., Waszkiel, D. (2006) Prosthetic status and needs of HIV positive subjects. *Adv. Med. Sci.*, 51(1): 106-109.

Corrigan, P. W., Watson, A. C. (2002) The paradox of self-stigma and mental illness. *Clinical Psychol. Sci. Prac.*, 9(1):35-53.

Dougall, A., Martinez Pereira, F., Molina, G., Eschevins, C., Daly, B., Faulks, D. (2018) Identifying common factors of functioning, participation and environment amongst adults requiring specialist oral health care using the International Classification of Functioning, disability and health. *PLoS ONE*, 13(7): e0199781.

Emlet, C. (2005) Measuring stigma in older and younger adults with HIV/AIDS: an analysis of an HIV stigma scale and initial exploration of subscales. *Res. Soc. Work Pract.*, 15(4):291-300.

Fleming, T. R., Cohen, M. S., Chen, Y. Q., McCauley, M., Gamble, T., Hosseinipour, M. C., Kumarasamy, N., Hakim, J. G., Grinsztejn, B., Godbole, S. V., Chariyalertsak, S., Santos, B. R., Mayer, K. H.,

Hoffman, I. F., Eshleman, S. H., Piwowar-Manning, E., Cottle, L., Zhang, X. C., Makhema, J., Mills, L. A., Panchia, R., Faesen, S., Eron, J., Gallant, J., Havlir, D., Swindells, S., Elharrar, V., Burns, D., Taha, T. E., Nielsen-Saines, K., Celentano, D. D., Essex, M., Hudelson, S. E., Redd, A. D., Pilotto, J. H. S. (2016) Antiretroviral Therapy for the Prevention of HIV-1 Transmission. *JAIDS*, 375: 830-839.

Gazhva, S. I., Stepanyan, T. B., Goryacheva, T. P. (2014) Prevalence of dental diseases of the oral mucosa and their diagnosis. *International Journal of Applied and Basic Research*, 5(1): 41-44.

Gesesew, H. A., Tesfay Gebremedhin, A., Demissie, T. D., Kerie, M. W., Sudhakar, M., Mwanri, L. (2017) Significant association between perceived HIV related stigma and late presentation for HIV/AIDS care in low and middle-income countries: A systematic review and meta-analysis. *PLoS ONE*, 12(3): e0173928.

Giuliani, M., Lajolo, C., Rezza, G., Arici, C., Babudieri, S., Grima, P., et al. (2005) Dental care and HIV-infected individuals: are they equally treated? *Community Dent. Oral Epidemiol.*, 33(6):447-453.

Hatzenbuehler, M., Phelan, J., Link, B. (2013) Stigma as a fundamental cause of population health inequalities. *Am. J. Public Health*, 103(5):813-821.

Ioannidi, E. A., Chernyavskaya, O. A., Kozyrev, O. A. (2013) Some ethical and legal aspects of the problem of providing medical care to people living with HIV/AIDS. *Bioethics*, 1: 41-46.

Kirsanova, S. V., Bazikyan, E. A., Gurevich, K. G., Fabrikant, E. G. (2007) Clinical and social characteristics of patients with partial absence of teeth and the introduction of quality of life criteria for evaluating the effectiveness of treatment. *Institute of Dentistry*, 4(37): 24-25.

Knuf, A., Epov, L. Yu. (2006) Stigma: Theory and Practice. *Knowledge. Understanding. Skill*, 2: 149-153.

Logie, C., Gadalla, T. (2009) Meta-analysis of health and demographic correlates of stigma towards people living with HIV. *AIDS Care*, 21(6): 742-753.

Mak, W. W., Poon, C. Y., Pun, L. Y., Cheung, S. F. (2007) Meta-analysis of stigma and mental health. *Soc. Sci. Med.*, 65(2):245-261.

Pokrovsky, V. V. (Ed.) (2013) *HIV infection and AIDS: national leadership.* Moscow: GEOTAR-Media.

Popova, T. G., Bazikyan, E. A., Pashinyan, G. A., Kamalyan, A. V., Kuraeva, E. Yu. (2008) On the criteria for expert assessment of adverse outcomes in the provision of dental implant care. *Forensic examination*, 51(2): 21-23.

Reznik, D. A. (2005) Oral manifestations of HIV disease. *Top. HIV Med.*, 13(5):143-148.

Research Report Moscow (2010) *People Living with HIV Stigma Index.* Доступно по ссылке [Available here]: www.stigmaindex.org/russian-federation (дата обращения: 01 февраля 2019 [Date of contact: February 01, 2019]).

Ruziev, M. M., Bandaev, I. S., Son, I. M., Raupov, F. O. (2018). The results of sociological studies to identify forms of stigmatization and discrimination against people living with HIV in Tajikistan. *Social aspects of public health*, 59(1): 7.

Safren, S. A., Mayer, K. H., Ou, S-S, McCauley, M., Grinsztejn, B., Hosseinipour, M. C., Kumarasamy, N., Gamble, T., Hoffman, I., Celentano, D., Chen, Y. Q., Cohen, M. S. (2015) Adherence to Early Antiretroviral Therapy: Results from HPTN 052, A Phase III, Multinational Randomized Trial of ART to Prevent HIV-1 Sexual Transmission in Serodiscordant Couples. *Journal of Acquired Immune Deficiency Syndromes*, 69(2): 234-240.

Stutterheim, S. E., Pryor, J. B., Bos, A. E., Hoogendijk, R., Muris, P., Schaalma, H. P. (2009) HIV-related stigma and psychological distress: the harmful effects of specific stigma manifestations in various social settings. *AIDS*, 23(17): 2353-2357.

UNAIDS (2005) *HIV Stigma, Discrimination, and Human Rights Violations: Case Studies of Successful Programs.* Available at the link: http://data.unaids.org/publications/irc-pub06/jc999-hrviolations_ru.pdf (access date: February 10, 2019).

United Nations Development Program (UNDP) (2008) *Living with HIV in Eastern Europe and the CIS: consequences of social exclusion*. Available at the link: www.unrussia.ru/sites/default/files/doc/AIDS%20russ_7_12_2008.pdf (access date: February 10, 2019).

Watt, R. G., Heilmann, A., Listl, S., Peres, M. A. (2016) London Charter on Oral Health Inequalities. *J. Dent. Res.*, 95(3):245-247.

World Health Organization (2010) *Equity, social determinants and public health programs*. Available at the link: http://apps.who.int/iris/bitstream/handle/10665/44289/9789241563970_eng.pdf?sequen== (access date: February 10, 2019).

World Health Organization (2003) *World Health Organization Report*. Available at the link: www.who.int/oral_health/publications/world-oral-health-report-2003/en/ (appeal date: February 10, 2019).

In: HIV/AIDS
Editor: Ethel K. Hebert

ISBN: 978-1-53617-923-1
© 2020 Nova Science Publishers, Inc.

Chapter 3

MANAGEMENT OF HEPATITIS C VIRUS IN PATIENTS COINFECTED WITH HIV

Soha Freidy and Olga M. Klibanov[*]

Wingate University School of Pharmacy, Wingate University,
Wingate, NC, US

ABSTRACT

Hepatitis C virus (HCV) is a bloodborne disease transmitted via direct contact with HCV infected blood. Human immunodeficiency virus (HIV) can be transmitted through direct contact with HIV infected blood. Due to their common route of transmission, HCV infection is prevalent among HIV patients. About 62-80% of HIV patients are coinfected with HCV according to the Center for Disease Control and Prevention (CDC). The efficacy and safety profile of modern HCV therapy [i.e., direct-acting antivirals (DAA)] is similar among coinfected patients and mono-infected patients. However, HCV/HIV coinfected patients require continuous monitoring due to drug-drug interaction with DAAs and antiretroviral drugs. Treating HCV infection while maintaining adequate HIV suppression could be challenging. For this reason, the American Association for the Study of Liver Diseases (AASLD) and the Infectious

---
[*] Corresponding Author's Email: o.klibanov@wingate.edu.

Disease Society of America (IDSA) published recommendations for managing and treating coinfected patients. This chapter will review the recommended treatment for chronic HCV infection with HIV coinfection, focusing on the pharmacokinetics and pharmacology of drug-drug interactions between antiretroviral therapy and DAAs.

INTRODUCTION

Overview of Hepatitis C Virus (HCV)

Hepatitis C virus (HCV) is a bloodborne virus which can cause chronic and acute infections. Acute infections are rarely symptomatic and usually lead to chronic infection in 85% of patients. Chronic infections can cause liver cirrhosis, hepatocellular carcinoma (HCC) and a need for liver transplantation. HCV is the one of the major causes of death globally [1]. The World Health Organization (WHO) estimates 71 million infected with chronic HCV globally. HCV infections occur worldwide, with the highest prevalence in the Middle East (2.3%) and European regions (1.5%) according to 2015 estimates [2]. The Center of Disease Control and Prevention (CDC) estimates that 3.9 million persons are infected with HCV without knowledge of their HCV status. Most of these patients serve as a source of transmission of HCV virus [3].

HCV is a single RNA virus that infect the liver and replicate within the hepatocytes. HCV continuously mutates due to the deficiency in proofreading polymerase [4]. Six genotypes (GT) have been identified for HCV virus (1-6) and subtypes (1a and 1b). The most common genotype in the United States is GT1 and accounts for 75% of patients [5, 6]. HCV consists of core that surrounds the RNA genome and viral envelope which plays an important role for viral entry [7].

Risk Factors for HCV

HCV is transmitted through direct contact with blood, such as injection drug use with shared injection equipment, blood transfusion with infected blood or blood product, and sexual practices that lead to blood exposure (men who have sex with men, especially who are HIV infected or those who are taking pre-exposure prophylaxis against HIV). In the United States, persons who inject drugs (PWID) account for 60% of HCV infections [2].

HCV/HIV Coinfection Risk Factors

Due to modes of transmission, HCV/HIV coinfection is common. According to the CDC, about 25% of HIV patients are coinfected with HCV. Moreover, 75% of HIV persons who inject drugs are coinfected with HCV [3, 8]. Despite the effective antiretroviral therapy (ART), HCV/HIV coinfection is associated with faster liver disease progression and a higher liver disease - associated mortality. HIV coinfection can increase HCV replication, decrease HCV clearance and hinder a response to therapy with direct acting antivirals (DAAs). The mechanism of liver damage is not well-understood; however, HCV/HIV coinfected cells have higher HCV RNA and HIV-1 RNA levels than monoinfected cells. Some data suggest that coinfection may intensify hepatocyte apoptosis which accelerates liver fibrosis [9].

MANAGEMENT OF HCV/HIV COINFECTED PATIENTS

Screening

The CDC estimates that half of the chronically infected patients with HCV don't know they are infected [10]. For this reason, the American Association for the Study of Liver disease (AASLD) and Infectious Diseases Society of America (IDSA) recommend screening patients according to the risk behaviors like injection drug use, risk conditions and circumstance like persons with HIV infections, and risks of exposure like persons on long-term hemodialysis (Table 1) [10, 11]. A one-time routine screening is recommended to all individuals 18 years of age and older to rule out infections, and annual HCV testing for all persons who inject drugs and for men with HIV infection who have unprotected sex with men. In addition, screening for hepatitis B virus (HBV) antigens (HBsAg) is recommended for currently HCV infected patients. Detection of HBsAg requires monitoring due to the risk of HBV activation during therapy with DAAs [11].

Diagnosis and Pretreatment Laboratory Recommendations

Screening for HCV antibodies is the initial step in HCV testing. Detection of HCV antibodies indicates that the person is currently infected (acute or chronic) or was previously infected and either cleared the infection spontaneously or cured with HCV medications in the past. If the HCV antibody test is positive, HCV RNA testing is recommended to confirm current active infection [11].

Treating HCV is not only beneficial for HCV patients, but it also helps eradicate HCV globally by reducing transmission. The goal of treatment of HCV infection is to reduce mortality and liver-related comorbidities. This goal is achieved through a sustained virologic response (SVR). SVR is achieved when patients' assay remains undetectable for HCV RNA for ≥ 12 weeks after treatment completion. Initiation of HCV treatment is recommended for all HCV infected patients, except patients with a short life expectancy that will not change with HCV treatment and those in need of liver transplantation. Patients starting on DAA therapy should be monitored before treatment, during treatment and post-treatment.

The following laboratories are recommended prior to therapy with DAAs and within 6 months of initiation of DAAs: complete blood count (CBC), international normalized ratio (INR), hepatic function panel, estimated glomerular normalized filtration rate (eGFR), quantitative HCV RNA, HCV genotype and subtype. In addition, assessments of HBV infection, HIV infection, extent of liver disease, and potential drug-drug interactions should be performed [11].

Table 1. Recommended populations to screen for HCV [11]

Anyone born between 1945 and 1965
Past use of active use of injection drug use
Coinfection with HIV
Received blood transfusion or organ transplantation before 1992 or clotting factors before 1987
Patient on hemodialysis or been on hemodialysis
Sexual partners of HCV-positive patients

During treatment with DAAs, which typically lasts 8-12 weeks in uncomplicated cases, patients should follow-up with their providers monthly to be evaluated for medication adherence and to have basic laboratory assessments performed. After completion of therapy, patients should return in 12 weeks to assess their HCV RNA. If the HCV RNA level is under the level of detection, then the patient is considered to have achieved SVR12 (i.e., cure). In non-cirrhotic patients who achieve SVR, no further HCV monitoring is needed; they should receive standard of care as if they have never been infected with HCV. However, if the patient has advanced fibrosis (F3) or cirrhosis (F4), it is recommended that they have liver ultrasound evaluations every 6 months to monitor for HCC [11].

HCV Medications: Direct Acting Antivirals (DAAs)

Modern HCV therapy consists of DAAs. These medications work by inhibiting viral replication through interfering with non-structural (NS) proteins essential for HCV replication. DAAs with different mechanisms of action are typically manufactured as fixed-dose combination tablets and are administered as a simple once-daily regimen. The most commonly used DAA therapies include ledipasvir/sofosbuvir (Harvoni®), sofosbuvir/velpatasvir (Epclusa®), sofosbuvir/velpatasvir/voxilaprevir (Vosevi®), glecaprevir/pibrentasvir (Mavyret®), and elbasvir/grazoprevir (Zepatier®). Table 2 outlines the various DAAs and their mechanisms of action.

Table 2. Mechanisms of action of DAAs [12-16]

Direct Acting Antiviral	Mechanism of Action
Ledipasvir Velpatasvir Pibrentasvir Elbasvir	*NS5A inhibitors*: inhibit HCV NS5A protein required for viral replication
Sofosbuvir	*NS5B inhibitor*: HCV BS5B RNA-dependent RNA polymerase, competes with the natural substrates for binding to the catalytic site of RNA polymerase and termination of the RNA chain.
Glecaprevir Grazoprevir Voxilaprevir	*NS3/4A protease inhibitors*: inhibit HCV NS3/4A protease enzyme which is necessary for the cleavage of HCV encoded polyproteins; NS3, NS4A, NS4B, NS5A, and NS5B

Clinical Trial Data in Patients with HCV/HIV Coinfection

Despite the high prevalence of HCV in the HIV infected population, few DAA trials have been performed in this population (Table 3). Ledipasvir/sofosbuvir (LDV/SOF) was evaluated in two clinical trials in HCV/HIV coinfected patients. The ERADICATE trial was a small pilot study that demonstrated a SVR12 rate of 98% with LDV/SOF and good tolerability, with the most commonly reported adverse effects of headaches and fatigue [17]. ION-4 was a large phase 3 multicenter study in the HCV/HIV coinfected population, demonstrating a 96% SVR12 rate that was similar in patients with or without compensated cirrhosis [18]. Both trials did not report significant change in HIV-1 RNA or CD4 counts. The results of these trials suggest that LDV/SOF is safe and effective for HCV/HIV coinfected patients taking LDV/SOF [17, 18].

Sofosbuvir/velpatasvir (SOF/VEL) was evaluated in a phase 3 ASTRAL-5 study that enrolled 106 HCV/HIV coinfected patients with genotypes 1-4. SVR12 was achieved in 95% of patients and all 19 patients with cirrhosis achieved SVR12 [19].

Glecaprevir/pibrentasvir (GLE/PIB) was evaluated in a phase 3 EXPEDITION-2 trial that enrolled 153 HCV/HIV coinfected patients with genotypes 1-6. Patients without cirrhosis received 8 weeks of GLE/PIB and those with cirrhosis received 12 weeks of therapy. SVR12 was achieved in 98% of patients; 100% in patients without cirrhosis achieved SRV12 and 93% with cirrhosis achieved SVR12. Most common adverse events were fatigue, headache and nausea [20].

Table 3. Clinical trials with DAAs in HCV/HIV coinfected patients [17-23]

Study	Population	Intervention	SVR12	Comments
ERADICATE [17] Ph2b, SC, UC, OL, NR	GT 1 without cirrhosis (n = 50)	LDV/SOF x 12 wks.	98%	Small pilot study
ION-4 [18] Ph3, MC, OL	GT 1 and 4 with and without compensated cirrhosis (n = 335)	LDV/SOF x 12 wks	96%	SVR rates were similar in non-cirrhotics vs. cirrhotics
ASTRAL-5 [19] Ph3, OL	GT 1-4 with or without compensated cirrhosis (n = 106)	SOF/VEL x 12 wks	95%	All patients with cirrhosis (n = 19) achieved SVR12
EXPEDITION-2 [20] Ph3, MC, OL	GT 1-6 with or without compensated cirrhosis (n=153)	GLE/PIB x 8 wks in non-cirrhotics or 12 wks in cirrhotics	98%	Prior treatment with SOF or IFN did not affect SVR12 rates
C-EDGE COINFECTION [21] Ph3, UC, NR	GT 1, 4, 6 with or without compensated cirrhosis (n=218)	ELB/GRZ x 12 wks	96%	All patients with cirrhosis (N=35) achieved SVR12
RESOLVE [22] Ph2b, MC, OL	GT 1 with prior DAA failure (n = 77)	SOF/VEL/VOX x 12 wks	90.9% overall; 82.4% in HIV coinfected	Only 17 patients were coinfected with HIV. HIV did not impact SVR12 rate
Veterans Affairs (VA) [23] OB, ITT cohort	GT1 with and without cirrhosis (n = 757)	LDV/SOF +/- RBV or OPrD +/- RBV x 12 wks	90.9%	SVR12 was higher in non-cirrhotics vs. cirrhotics (92% vs 86%)

Ph: phase; SVR12: sustained virologic response 12 weeks after completion of therapy (i.e., "cure"); OB: observational; ITT: intention-to-treat; LDV/SOF: ledipasvir/sofosbuvir; RBV: ribavirin; OPrD: ombitasvir/paritaprevir/ritonavir/dasabuvir; SC: single center; UC: uncontrolled; OL: open label; NR: nonrandomized; MC: multi-center; SOF/VEL: sofosbuvir/velpatasvir; GLE/PIB: glecaprevir/pibrentasvir; NR: non-randomized; ELB/GRZ: elbasvir/grazoprevir; SOF/VEL/VOX: sofosbuvir/velpatasvir/voxilaprevir.

Elbasvir/grazoprevir (ELB/GRZ) was assessed in the C-EDGE COINFECTION multicenter study that included 218 HCV/HIV coinfected patients with GT 1, 4, or 6. SVR12 was achieved in 96% of patients. All 35 patients with compensated cirrhosis achieved SVR12. Most common adverse effects were fatigue, headache, and nausea [21].

Data with sofosbuvir/velpatasvir/voxilaprevir (SOF/VEL/VOX) in the HCV/HIV coinfected population are limited. The RESOLVE study enrolled 77 patients with genotype 1 and a history of prior DAA failure, of whom 17 were coinfected with HIV. SVR12 was 90.9% in the overall population and 82.4% in HIV coinfected patients. In this small trial HIV coinfection did not significantly impact the SVR12 rate [22].

Veterans Affairs (VA) did a large "real life" observational study in the HCV/HIV coinfected population with genotype 1 infection. The purpose of the study is to observe the effectiveness of ledipasvir/sofosbuvir (LDV/SOF) +/- ribavirin or ombitasvir/paritaprevir/ritonavir plus dasabuvir in this patient population. SVR rates were 90.9% overall, liver cirrhosis was associated with lower SVR rates [23].

These data suggest that the efficacy and safety of DAAs in the HCV/HIV coinfected population is similar to the data in HCV monoinfected patients. Therefore, AASLD and IDSA guidelines recommend similar treatment protocols for HCV/HIV coinfected patients as for HCV mono-infected patients, with some differences in therapy durations for certain DAAs [11].

Recommended First Line Therapy

Recommended initial treatment regimens for HCV-infected treatment-naïve patients with and without compensated cirrhosis are described in Tables 4 and 5, respectively.

Patients with decompensated liver cirrhosis should be referred to a specialist to manage their HCV therapy, preferably at a liver transplant center. The management of patients with a history of prior failures to HCV medications is beyond the scope of this chapter; the AASLD HCV guidelines should be consulted on how to treat these more complicated patient populations [11].

Table 4. Recommended initial regimens for patients without cirrhosis [11]

Genotype	Treatment	Duration
1	elbasvir/grazoprevir	12 weeks
	glecaprevir/pibrentasvir	8 weeks
	ledipasvir/sofosbuvir	12 weeks 8 weeks (if HIV uninfected and HCV RNA level <6 million IU/mL)
	sofosbuvir/velpatasvir	12 weeks
2, 3	glecaprevir/pibrentasvir	8 weeks
	sofosbuvir/velpatasvir	12 weeks
4	glecaprevir/pibrentasvir	8 weeks
	ledipasvir/sofosbuvir	12 weeks
	sofosbuvir/velpatasvir	12 weeks
	elbasvir/grazoprevir	12 weeks
5, 6	glecaprevir/pibrentasvir	8 weeks (12 weeks if HIV-infected)
	ledipasvir/sofosbuvir	12 weeks
	sofosbuvir/velpatasvir	12 weeks

Table 5. Recommended initial regimens for patients with compensated liver cirrhosis [11]

Genotype	Treatment	Duration
1	elbasvir/grazoprevir	12 weeks
	glecaprevir/pibrentasvir	8 weeks (12 weeks if HIV-infected)
	ledipasvir/sofosbuvir	12 weeks
	sofosbuvir/velpatasvir	12 weeks
2, 3	glecaprevir/pibrentasvir	8 weeks (12 weeks if HIV-infected)
	sofosbuvir/velpatasvir	12 weeks
4	glecaprevir/pibrentasvir	8 weeks (12 weeks if HIV-infected)
	ledipasvir/sofosbuvir	12 weeks
	sofosbuvir/velpatasvir	12 weeks
	elbasvir/grazoprevir	12 weeks
5, 6	glecaprevir/pibrentasvir	8 weeks (12 weeks if HIV-infected)
	ledipasvir/sofosbuvir	12 weeks
	sofosbuvir/velpatasvir	12 weeks

DAAs and Drug-Drug Interactions (DDIs)

DAAs have complex metabolism and DDI profiles. SOF is a prodrug that is converted to its active form that inhibits the NS5B RNA dependent polymerase. LDV/SOF is a substrate of P-gp and breast cancer resistant protein (BCRB) while the active metabolite of sofosbuvir is not. Co-administration with P-gp inducers is not recommended due to reduction of LDV/SOF plasma concentrations and reduced therapeutic effect [12].

SOF/VEL are substrates of the P-gp and BCRB. Co-administration with P-gp inducers is not recommended due to reduction of SOF/VEL plasma concentration and reduce therapeutic effect. Velpatasvir is also metabolized by CYP3A4, CYP2C8 and CYP2B6 and is a substrate and inhibitor of P-gp and BCRP [13].

GLE/PIB are inhibitors and substrates of the P-gp, BCRB and organic anion transporting polypeptide (OATP) 1B1/3. GLE/PIB may increase the concentrations of drugs that are substrates for these transporters. In addition, GLE/PIB concentrations may be increased by coadministration with transport inhibitors and decreased with coadministration of transport inducers. GLE/PIB are also weak inhibitors of CYP3A, CYP1A2, and uridine glucuronosyltransferase (UGT) [15].

ELB/GRZ are substrates of CYP 3A4 and P-gp; coadministration with CYP3A4 and P-gp inducers such as efavirenz is not recommended. GRZ is a substrate of liver uptake transporter OATP1B1, coadministration with OATP1B1 inhibitors can increase risk of hepatotoxicity due to the increase in GRZ plasma concentrations [16].

VOX is a substrate of P-gp, OATP, CYP 3A4, CYP 1A2, CYP2C8. VOX inhibits P-gp, OATP and BCRP. Drugs that induce the P-gp and/or potent inducers of CYP2B6, CYP2C8, or CYP3A4 may decrease the plasma concentrations of SOF/VEL/VOX and put the patient at risk of DAA therapeutic failure [14].

Assessment DDIs is recommended for all patients before starting DAA therapy. DDIs can be assessed using AASLD/IDSA guidelines [11], the University of Liverpool HEP Drug Interactions website [24], or other drug information sources. It is important to have a comprehensive list of all medications including over the counter (OTC) medications and herbal products. For example, some DAAs need an acidic environment to be absorbed; therefore, taking OTC acid reducers can lower their bioavailability, putting the patient at risk of DAA treatment failure. Table 6 describes the interactions between DAAs and some of the commonly used medications. Medications that are bolded should be avoided; those that are italicized should be used with caution and monitoring; the ones in plain text are safe to co-administer.

Table 6. Drug-drug interactions between DAAs and commonly used drugs [11]

	LDV/SOF	SOF/VEL	GLE/PIB	ELB/GRZ	SOF/VEL/VOX
Acid-reducing agents	*Antacid* *H2RA* *PPI*	*Antacid* *H2RA* *PPI*	Antacid H2RA PPI	*Antacid* *H2RA* *PPI*	*Antacid* *H2RA* *PPI*
Statins	Rosuvastatin *Atorvastatin* *Fluvastatin* *Lovastatin* *Pitavastatin* *Pravastatin* *Simvastatin*	*Rosuvastatin* *Atorvastatin* *Fluvastatin* *Lovastatin* *Simvastatin*	**Simvastatin** Atorvastatin Lovastatin *Fluvastatin* *Rosuvastatin* *Pitavastatin*	*Rosuvastatin* *Atorvastatin* *Fluvastatin* *Lovastatin* *Simvastatin*	Rosuvastatin **Pitavastatin** *Atorvastatin* *Fluvastatin* *Lovastatin* *Pravastatin* *Simvastatin*
Anticonvulsants	**Carbamazepine** **Phenytoin**	**Carbamazepine** **Phenytoin**	**Carbamazepine** **Phenytoin**	**Carbamazepine** **Phenytoin**	**Carbamazepine** **Phenytoin**
Antiarrhythmic	**Amiodarone** *Digoxin*	**Amiodarone** *Digoxin*	*Amiodarone* *Digoxin*	*Amiodarone*	*Amiodarone* *Digoxin*
Anticoagulants and antiplatelets agents	*Apixaban* *Dabigatran* *Edoxaban* *Rivaroxaban* *Ticagrelor* *Warfarin*	*Apixaban* *Dabigatran* *Edoxaban* *Rivaroxaban* *Ticagrelor* *Warfarin*	**Dabigatran** *Apixaban* *Edoxaban* *Rivaroxaban* *Ticagrelor* *Warfarin*	*Apixaban* *Dabigatran* *Edoxaban* *Rivaroxaban* *Ticagrelor* *Warfarin*	**Dabigatran** **Edoxaban** *Apixaban* *Rivaroxaban* *Ticagrelor* *Warfarin*
Herbal	**St. John's wort**	**St. John's wort**	**St. John's wort**	**St. John's wort**	**St. John's wort**

LDV/SOF: ledipasvir/sofosbuvir; SOF/VEL: sofosbuvir/velpatasvir; GLE/PIB: glecaprevir/pibrentasvir; ELB/GRZ: elbasvir/grazoprevir; SOF/VEL/VOX: sofosbuvir/velpatasvir/voxilaprevir; H2RA: histamine H$_2$ antagonist; PPIs: proton pump inhibitors.

In the HCV/HIV coinfected population, managing DDIs between DAAs and ART is the biggest challenge while maintaining adequate response to both therapies. Similar to DAAs, many of the HIV medications undergo complex metabolism pathways and have many potential DDIs associated with them. Special attention to potential DDIs between DAAs and ART should be given when HCV therapy is being initiated in coinfected patients [11]. Table 7 describes the interactions between DAAs and commonly used HIV medications.

Table 7. DDIs between DAAs and antiretrovirals [11]

HIV Drug Class	HIV Drug	LDV/SOF	SOF/VEL	GLE/PIB	GRZ/ELB	SOF/VEL/VOX
HIV Protease Inhibitors	Boosted atazanavir	Caution if also using with TDF	Caution if also using with TDF	Avoid	Avoid	Avoid
	Boosted darunavir	Caution if also using with TDF	Caution if also using with TDF	Avoid	Avoid	Use with caution; monitor therapy
	Boosted lopinavir	Caution if also using with TDF	Caution if also using with TDF	Avoid	Avoid	Avoid
NNRTIs	Doravirine	Safe to use	Safe to use	Safe to use	Safe to use	Safe to use
	Efavirenz	Safe to use	Avoid	Avoid	Avoid	Avoid
	Rilpivirine	Safe to use	Safe to use	Safe to use	Safe to use	Safe to use
	Etravirine	Safe to use	Avoid	Avoid	Avoid	Avoid
Integrase Inhibitors	Bictegravir	Safe to use	Safe to use	Safe to use	Safe to use	Safe to use
	Cobicistat-boosted elvitegravir	Avoid if also using with TDF in patients with eGFR <60 mL/min	Avoid if also using with TDF in patients with eGFR <60 mL/min	Avoid if also using with TDF in patients with eGFR <60 mL/min	Avoid	Avoid if also using with TDF in patients with eGFR <60 mL/min
	Dolutegravir	Safe to use	Safe to use	Safe to use	Safe to use	Safe to use
	Raltegravir	Safe to use	Safe to use	Safe to use	Safe to use	Safe to use
NRTIs	Abacavir	Safe to use	Safe to use	Safe to use	Safe to use	Safe to use
	Emcitabine	Safe to use	Safe to use	Safe to use	Safe to use	Safe to use
	Lamivudine	Safe to use	Safe to use	Safe to use	Safe to use	Safe to use
	Tenofovir disoproxil fumarate	Avoid in patients with eGFR <60 mL/min	Avoid in patients with eGFR <60 mL/min	Safe to use	Safe to use	Avoid in patients with eGFR <60 mL/min
	Tenofovir alafenamide	Safe to use	Safe to use	Safe to use	Safe to use	Safe to use

LDV/SOF: ledipasvir/sofosbuvir; SOF/VEL: sofosbuvir/velpatasvir; GLE/PIB: glecaprevir/pibrentasvir; ELB/GRZ: elbasvir/grazoprevir; SOF/VEL/VOX: sofosbuvir/velpatasvir/voxilaprevir; TDF: tenofovir disoproxil fumarate.

CONCLUSION

A high proportion of HIV-infected individuals are also coinfected with HCV. Whereas in the past, HCV was very difficult to treat in this population and had very low success rates, the novel DAAs have revolutionized treatment of HCV in these patients. DAA regimens are very well tolerated, can be given as a very low pill burden regimen for a very short period of time (8-12 weeks) and can result in HCV cure in over 95% of patients, regardless of the presence of HIV coinfection. One of the main concerns in the HCV/HIV coinfected population with DAAs is the potential for DDIs. Clinicians treating this population must be diligent in screening for DDIs in these patients to ensure minimal adverse outcomes and optimal HCV cure rates. Many resources are available and should be utilized for DDI screening. HCV infection in most HCV/HIV coinfected patients can now be treated and cured successfully.

REFERENCES

[1] Petruzziello, A., S. Marigliano, G. Loquercio, A. Cozzolino, and C. Cacciapuoti. 2016. "Global epidemiology of hepatitis C virus infection: An up-date of the distribution and circulation of hepatitis C virus genotypes." *World J. Gastroenterol.* 22: 7824-40.

[2] The World Health Organization (WHO). *Hepatitis C.* Accessed March 15, 2020. https://www.who.int/news-room/fact-sheets/detail/hepatitis-c.

[3] Centers for Disease Control and Prevention (CDC). "HIV and Viral Hepatitis". Accessed March 15, 2020. https://www.cdc.gov/hiv/pdf/library/factsheets/hiv-viral-hepatitis.pdf.

[4] Kanto, T., and N. Hayashi. 2006. "Immunopathogenesis of hepatitis C virus infection: multifaceted strategies subverting innate and adaptive immunity." *Intern. Med.* 45: 183-91.

[5] Germer, J. J., J. N. Mandrekar, J. L. Bendel, P. S. Mitchell, and J. D. Yao. 2011. "Hepatitis C virus genotypes in clinical specimens tested at a national reference testing laboratory in the United States." *J. Clin. Microbiol.* 49: 3040-3.

[6] Guss, D., J. Sherigar, P. Rosen, and S. R. Mohanty. 2018. "Diagnosis and Management of Hepatitis C Infection in Primary Care Settings". *J. Gen. Intern. Med.* 33: 551-57.

[7] Dubuisson, J., and F. L. Cosset. 2014. "Virology and cell biology of the hepatitis C virus life cycle: an update." *J. Hepatol.* 61: S3-S13.

[8] Platt, L., P. Easterbrook, E. Gower, B. McDonald, K. Sabin, C. McGowan, et al. 2016. "Prevalence and burden of HCV co-infection in people living with HIV: a global systematic review and meta-analysis." *Lancet Infect. Dis.* 16: 797-808.

[9] Ganesan, M., L. Y. Poluektova, K. K. Kharbanda, and N. A. Osna. 2019. "Human immunodeficiency virus and hepatotropic viruses co-morbidities as the inducers of liver injury progression." *World J. Gastroenterol.* 25: 398-410.

[10] Centers for Disease Control and Prevention (CDC). *Hepatitis C Prevalence Estimates 2013-2016*. Accessed March 15, 2020. https://www.cdc.gov/nchhstp/newsroom/2018/hepatitis-c-prevalence-estimates.html.

[11] AASLD-IDSA. *Recommendations for testing, managing, and treating hepatitis C*. Accessed March 15, 2020. http://www.hcvguidelines.org.

[12] *HARVONI [package insert]*. Foster City, CA: Gilead Sciences; 2019.

[13] *EPCLUSA [package insert]*. Foster City, CA: Gilead Sciences; 2019.

[14] *VOSEVI [package insert]*. Foster City, CA: Gilead Sciences; 2019.

[15] *MAVYRET [package insert]*. North Chicago, IL: AbbVie Inc.; 2020.

[16] *ZEPATIER [package insert]*. Whitehouse Station, NJ: Merck & Co., Inc.; 2019.

[17] Osinusi, A., K. Townsend, A. Kohli, A. Nelson, C. Seamon, E. G. Meissner, et al. 2015. "Virologic response following combined ledipasvir and sofosbuvir administration in patients with HCV genotype 1 and HIV co-infection." *JAMA* 313: 1232-9.

[18] Naggie, S., C. Cooper, M. Saag, K. Workowski, P. Ruane, W. J. Towner, et al. 2015. "Ledipasvir and Sofosbuvir for HCV in Patients Coinfected with HIV-1." *N. Engl. J. Med.* 373: 705-13.

[19] Wyles, D., N. Brau, S. Kottilil, E. S. Daar, P. Ruane, K. Workowski, et al. 2017. "Sofosbuvir and Velpatasvir for the Treatment of Hepatitis C Virus in Patients Coinfected With Human Immunodeficiency Virus Type 1: An Open-Label, Phase 3 Study." *Clin. Infect. Dis.* 65: 6-12.

[20] Rockstroh, J. K., K. Lacombe, R. M. Viani, C. Orkin, D. Wyles, A. F. Luetkemeyer, et al. 2018. "Efficacy and Safety of Glecaprevir/Pibrentasvir in Patients Coinfected With Hepatitis C Virus and Human Immunodeficiency Virus Type 1: The EXPEDITION-2 Study." *Clin. Infect. Dis.* 67: 1010-17.

[21] Rockstroh, J. K., M. Nelson, C. Katlama, J. Lalezari, J. Mallolas, M. Bloch, et al. 2015. "Efficacy and safety of grazoprevir (MK-5172) and elbasvir (MK-8742) in patients with hepatitis C virus and HIV co-infection (C-EDGE CO-INFECTION): a non-randomised, open-label trial." *Lancet HIV* 2: e319-27.

[22] Wilson, E., E. Covert, J. Hoffmann, E. Comstock, B. Emmanuel, L. Tang, et al. 2019. "A pilot study of safety and efficacy of HCV retreatment with sofosbuvir/velpatasvir/voxilaprevir in patients with or without HIV (resolve study)." *J. Hepatol.* 71: 498-504.

[23] Bhattacharya, D., P. S. Belperio, T. A. Shahoumian, T. P. Loomis, M. B. Goetz, L. A. Mole, et al. 2017. "Effectiveness of All-Oral Antiviral Regimens in 996 Human Immunodeficiency Virus/Hepatitis C Virus Genotype 1-Coinfected Patients Treated in Routine Practice." *Clin. Infect. Dis.* 64: 1711-20.

[24] University of Liverpool. *HEP Drug Interactions.* Accessed March 16, 2020. https://www.hep-druginteractions.org.

In: HIV/AIDS
Editor: Ethel K. Hebert

ISBN: 978-1-53617-923-1
© 2020 Nova Science Publishers, Inc.

Chapter 4

PREVENTION OF HIV/AIDS AMONG YOUTH

Todd Mamutle Maja, D Litt et Phil (PhD)*
Department of Health Studies
University of South Africa, Pretoria, South Africa

ACRONYMS

AIDS	Acquired Immunodeficiency Syndrome
ANC	Antenatal Care
ART	Antiretroviral Treatment
A/YFS	Adolescent/Youth Friendly Services
CDC	Centers for Disease Prevention and Control
HIV	Human Immunodeficiency Syndrome
PEPFAR	Presidents' Emergency Plan for AIDS
PLWHA	People living with HIV/AIDS
RDT	Rapid Diagnostic Test
SRH	Sexual and Reproductive Health
SSA	Sub Saharan Africa

---

* Corresponding Author's Email: majatmm@gmail.com.

UNAIDS	United Nations AIDS
UNICEF	United Nations Children's Fund
VCT	Voluntary Counselling and Testing
VMMC	Voluntary Medical Male Circumcision
WHO	World Health Organization

1. Introduction

Young people become sexually active at an early age and succumb to self-destructive behaviours such as alcohol and drug abuse, multiple sexual partners and unprotected sex resulting in unintentional pregnancies and sexually transmitted infections including HIV/AIDS.

Over 30% of all new HIV infections globally are estimated to occur among youth aged 15-24 years. In addition, children infected at birth grow into adolescents who have to deal with their HIV positive status, totalling 5 million youth living with HIV/AIDS. The greatest burden of HIV among young people is in the sub-Saharan Africa (SSA) (UNAIDS: 2016; WHO 2014, 2015).

Almost half of the 15-19 year olds who are living with HIV in the world, live in six countries, namely South Africa, Nigeria, Kenya, India, Mozambique and Tanzania. While HIV incidence and HIV- related deaths have decreased in other populations, in SSA, HIV-related deaths among youth continue to rise. Focusing on young people is likely to be the most effective approach to confronting the epidemic, particularly in high prevalence countries.

This chapter highlights HIV preventative measures which entail biomedical, behavioural and structural interventions as well as innovative technological strategies supported by literature sources from previous studies to provide evidence-based arguments.

2. BIOMEDICAL INTERVENTION

Biomedical intervention incorporates antiretroviral therapy (ART) for prevention and treatment of HIV/AIDS, voluntary male circumcision, voluntary HIV counselling and testing and vaginal microbicides

2.1. Antiretroviral Therapy

The introduction of ART is a remarkable breakthrough in the fight against HIV/AIDS, leading to significant decreases in HIV-related morbidity and mortality. The expansion in availability of ART over the past two decades has actually made HIV infection into a manageable chronic condition. People living with HIV and AIDS (PLWHA) now live longer and healthy lives on treatment. UNAIDS (2016) estimates that the global coverage of ART reached 48% in 2015, resulting in a 26% decrease in annual HIV related deaths.

HIV attacks and destroys the infection fighting CD4 cells of the immune system. Loss of CD4 cells makes it hard for the body to fight infection and certain HIV related cancers. HIV medicines prevent HIV from multiplying, which reduces the amount of HIV in the body-viral load. Having less HIV in the body gives the immune system a chance to recover.

ART is the use of HIV medicines to treat HIV infection. Doctors recommend taking a combination of medications referred to as antiretroviral therapy (ART) for people diagnosed with HIV/AIDS. Different multitudes of HIV drugs are available to control the virus and each type of drug blocks the virus in different ways.

ART is recommended for anyone who has HIV regardless of CD4 T cell count. Although ART cannot cure HIV, it helps people with HIV live longer, healthier lives by keeping HIV under control.

2.1.1. Classes of Anti-HIV Drugs

Classes of Anti-HIV Drugs include:

- Nucleoside or nucleotide reverse transcriptose inhibitors, are faulty version of the building blocks that HIV needs to make copies of itself. These are Abacavir (Ziagen) and the combination drugs emtricitabine (tenofovir (Truvada), Descovy (tenovir alafenamide/emtricitabine) and lamivudine (Combivir).
- Non-nucleoside reverse transcriptase inhibitors (NNR TLS) turn off a protein needed by HIV to make copies of itself. Examples of these drugs include efavirenz (Sustiva), etravirine ((intelence) and nevirapine (Veramune).
- Protease inhibitors (Pls) inactivate HIV protease, another protein that HIV needs to make copies of itself. Example include atazanavir (Reyataz), darunavir.
- Previstaf, osamprenavir (Lexiva) and indinas (Crixivan).
- Entry or fusion inhibitors. Tblock HIV's entry into CD4 T cells. Examples include enfuvirtide (Fuzen) and maraviroc (Selzentry).
- Intergrase inhibitors work by disabling s protein called intergrase, whichHIV uses to insrt its generic material into CD4 T cells, naltegravir is a typical example (Del Romero, Castilla, Hernando, Rodriquez & Garcia, 2010; Marco, Ajay, Nathan & Meg, 2019).

2.1.2. Commencement of Treatment

Everyone diagnosed with HIV infection regardless of CD4 T cell count should be offered antiviral medication as soon as possible.
HIV therapy is particularly important for the following when:

- Having severe symptoms;
- An opportunistic infection;
- CD4 T cell count is under 350;
- Pregnant;
- Having HIV related kidney disease;
- Being treated for hepatitis B or C.

2.1.3. Benefits of Taking HIV Medication as Prescribed

Benefits of taking HIV medication consistently far outweighs any risks. In his study on 'Massive benefits of ARV therapy in Africa', Vermund (2014), highlights the role played by PEPFAR and the Global fund in supporting priority countries impacted by HIV. The author pinpoints how millions of PLWHA's lives were saved since the introduction of ART. A total number of 6 million persons, mostly in the SSA among the 10 million persons were estimated to have begun ART as at 2013, with special reference to South Africa since implementation of ART medication in 2004. South Africa's aggregate benefits from ART from 2004 to 2011 (8years) are commensurate with the considerable benefits reported previously for the United States (US) from 1989 to 2003, that is,15 years (Vermund, 2006; Walensky, Paltiel, Losina et al., 2006). Other benefits of ART medication include: allows HIV medications to reduce the amount of HIV in person's body, helps to keep one's immune system stronger and better able to fight infections, reduces the risk of passing HIV to others and helps to prevent drug resistance.

2.1.4. Commonly Reported Side Effects of ART

HIV treatment plans may involve taking several pills at specific times daily for the rest of the person's life. Each medication has its own unique side effects. Some of the treatment's side effects include:

- Nausea and vomiting
- Diarrhoea
- Difficulty in sleeping
- Dry mouth
- Abnormal cholesterol levels
- Headache
- Rash
- Dizziness
- Fatigue
- Weakened bones

- Break down of muscle tissue
- Pain (Marco et al., 2019).

2.1.5. Adverse Effects of ART

When selecting an ARV regimen, clinicians must consider potential adverse effects and the individual's comorbidities, concomitant medications and prior history of drug tolerances to minimize the adverse effects. Factors that may predispose individuals to adverse effects of ARV medications include:

- Concomitant use of medications with overlapping and toxicities;
- Comorbid conditions that increase the risk of adverse effects, for example, underlying liver disease from alcohol use, coinfection with viral hepatitis, and or liver steatosis may increase the risk of hepatotoxicity when efavirenz or protease inhibitors are used.
- Certain ARVs may exacerbate pre-existing conditions such as psychiatric conditions being worsened by efavirenz, rilpivirine and infrequently by integrace strand transfer inhibitors.
- Drug-drug reactions may increase toxicities of ARV drugs or concomitant medications, for example, pharmacokinetic boosters-ritonavir or cobicistat are used or when isoniazid is used with efavirenz.
- Genetic factors that predispose patients to abacavir hypersensitivity reaction, neuro-psychiattric toxicity and atazanavir associated hyper-bilirubinema (den Brinker, Wit, Wertheim-van Dillen et al. 2000; Mallal, Phillips, Carosi et al., 2008).

2.1.6. Adherence to Antiretroviral Therapy

Adherence refers to a patient's ability to follow a treatment plan, take medications at prescribed times and frequencies and follow restrictions regarding food and other medications (WHO, 2010). Adherence to treatment plays a pivotal role in the success of medication provided for

PLWHA. ART has improved the quality of lives of PLWHA throughout the world.

A number of factors and barriers can result in non-adherence to HIV treatment. Studies on adherence and non-adherence to ART report:

- Research by Triphathi, Shukla, Argawal, Strivasta and Singh (2016) reveal that patients failed to adhere to treatment citing: busy with other things; felt sick or ill; had no money; forgot to bring medications when away from home; felt like the drug was harmful.
- Dewan, Lai & Rai (2010) found that 90% of participants in their study were adherent over four days and those who failed to adhere claimed being away from home and simply forgot to take their medication.
- Other systematic reviews of barriers to ART in developed and developing countries showed: fear to disclose HIV status; stigma; avoiding to take medication in public; side effects; using alternative HIV cure medicines; lack of continuous adherence education; judgemental attitudes of health care providers towards young people and transport problems (Bukenya et al., 2019; Dewan, Lai & Rai, 2010; WHO, 2010).

2.1.7. Conclusion

The large scale-up of ART, mainly in low and middle income countries has resulted in significant HIV prevention benefits in health as well as reductions in HIV-related morbidity and morbidity. PLWHA are urged to start with HIV treatment as soon as they are diagnosed for attaining viral suppression improving their own health. They should consult with the doctor or health care professionals and adhere to medication to maintain good health.

2.2. Voluntary Male Circumcision

Voluntary male circumcision refers to permanent or complete removal of the foreskin performed under local anaesthesia by several conventional or device-based surgical methods. The procedure is procured for medical reasons or as part of traditional, social and religious practices during early infancy, adolescence, youth and to adults. Voluntary male circumcision has been recommended by the WHO and UNAIDS in 2007 as an additional HIV prevention intervention in settings of high HIV prevalence.

2.2.1. Voluntary Medical Male Circumcision

VMMC was launched in fourteen priority countries as part of a comprehensive HIV prevention strategy and the programmes are recording annual output increases. An estimated number of 18,6 million cumulative medical circumcisions for HIV prevention were performed between 2008 and 2017 in priority countries of east and southern Africa. The annual number of voluntary medical circumcisions reached 4,4 million having averted 230,000 new infections by 2017 (WHO 2018). The WHO (2007) recommends a comprehensive package for Voluntary Medical Male Circumcision (VMMC) that includes HIV testing, safer sex education, STI management and condom distribution and promotion for integration into planning of comprehensive HIV prevention and Sexual Reproductive programmes.

Plotkin, Kuver, Curran et al., (2011) report that most clients accessing VMMC services are adolescents aged 10-19 years due to the following factors:

- Traditionally in circumcising communities, the social norm has been and continues to be for male circumcision to be part of rites of passage to adulthood.
- Service delivery models used to make VMMC more accessible to adolescents capitalize on school holidays coinciding with seasoned preferences in VMMC- seeking behaviours;
- Peer pressure is believed to be reinforcing VMMC service uptake.

However, structural factors such as limited clinic hours falling during school or work, lack of privacy, shame, prior negative experience with health care providers, limited sexual health education, fear of pain from the procedure and related injections have been reported as hindrances to VMMC (Kaufman, Smelyanskaya, Van Lith et al., 2016).

Removing the foreskin is associated with a variety of health benefits which include:

- Lower rates of urinary tract infections;
- Reduced risk of certain inflammations;
- Improved hygiene;
- Prevention of pathological conditions such as phimosis, which is common in uncircumcised men;
- Prevention of sexually transmitted infections including HIV/AIDS.

2.2.2. Traditional Male Circumcision

Traditional foreskin cutting has been widely performed for religious and cultural reasons often within two weeks of birth or at beginning of adolescence as a rite of passage to adulthood. It is regarded as a sacred and indispensable cultural rite intended to prepare initiates for the responsibilities of adulthood. Traditional male circumcision is mainly performed on adolescents or young men in a non-clinical setting by a traditional provider with no medical background.

This method is often associated with higher rates of complications and sometimes leading to death, than circumcision that is performed within the formal health care sector. Factors contributing to the harm caused include: traditional practitioners are often insufficiently trained to perform these surgeries; poor post-operative management such as binding the wound too tightly and traditional restrictions on drinking water leading to complications. According to Kepe (2010), from 1995 to 2005 in the Eastern Cape alone, 5,813 hospital admissions, 281 penile amputations and 342 deaths resulting from traditional circumcisions, were reported. In addition, scores of initiates experience medical complications and acquire treatment such as for septicaemia, gangrene, severe dehydration, genital mutilation and penile amputation (Behrens, 2014; Kepe, 2010; Ntombana, 2011). The right to keep the privilege may require that some of the customary aspects of practice need to change to prevent harm.

UNAIDS (2007) reports that trials in Kenya, Uganda and South Africa have all shown that male circumcision have significantly reduced man's risk of acquiring HIV by 50-60% after 21-24 months of follow up.

2.2.3. Conclusion

VMMC is a cost-effective biomedical intervention that has been proven to reduce the risk of female-to-male HIV transmission by up to 60% increasing to around 75% over time. Newly available circumcision devices play a role as an alternative to sutures and surgery that some men may prefer. The co-operation between the National Department of Health and Congress of Traditional leaders could play a major role in reducing complications resulting from traditional circumcisions.

2.3. Voluntary HIV Counselling and Testing

Voluntary HIV counselling and testing is a process by which an individual undergoes counselling, enabling him or her to make an informed choice about being tested for HIV. This decision must be entirely the choice of an individual and he or she must be assured that the process will be confidential.

The HIV test is a scientific test to show if a person has been infected with HIV and is usually done on a person's blood. Voluntary counselling and testing (VCT) has potential preventive effects on HIV transmission and serves as a gateway to most HIV/AIDS related services. VCT can change HIV-related sexual risk behaviours thereby reducing HIV-related risk and confirming its importance as an HIV prevention strategy.

VCT has long been regarded as an important intervention in the SSA offering a client-centered approach that addresses prevention of transmission between partners as well as between mother and child. Knowledge of HIV status is critical to achieve prevention and treatment goals.

2.3.1. Process of Voluntary Counselling and Testing

HIV counselling entails a face-to-face ***pre-test*** and ***post-test*** with individuals seeking to know their HIV status.

- *Pre-test counselling* aims at ensuring that individuals make informed decisions about whether to have HIV test or not. It further encourages individuals to explore the possible impact that having the test may have on them.
- *Post-test* counselling is conducted with an individual after the test during which the results are presented by the health care professional. Both these processes help people to cope better with results and more likely to look after their health and protect others from infection. Those testing HIV positive, ongoing counselling helps such individuals to accept their status and provides support including opportunities to talk to knowledgeable people who can help them understand their HIV status as well as guidance regarding any problems they may experience. A negative result offers a key opportunity to re-inforce the importance of safe and risk reducing behaviours.

UNAIDS (2014) recommends two types of HIV testing and Counselling for individuals; *client initiated* and *provider initiated testing* and counselling. Client initiated VCT involves individuals actively seeking HIV VCT at facilities that offer these services.

Provider initiated testing is recommended by health care providers to persons attending antenatal care services, where pregnant women diagnosed with HIV can benefit from receiving a package of HIV services as a way of expanding access to HIV VCT.

VCT should be voluntary and everyone being tested should give informed consent. This involves:

- Providing pre-test information on the purpose of testing and on treatment;
- Support should be available once the result is known;

- Ensuring understanding and respecting the individual's autonomy.
- Confidentiality must be respected, only health care providers should have a direct role and access to medical information

2.3.2. Potential Benefits of Voluntary Counselling and Testing

VCT has the potential to improve lives of people who might test HIV positive or negative. Their health benefits include:

- Improved health status through good nutritional advice and earlier access to care and treatment;
- Learning more about the virus and how it affects their body;
- Encourages individuals to look after their health and stay as healthy as possible;
- Get information and counselling around how to live positively with the virus;
- Learn to recognise the signs of opportunistic infections so as to be treated promptly;
- Find out what resources are available within communities to help people manage their HIV status;
- Find out about prophylactic drugs which help individuals from getting some opportunistic infections that are common with PLWHA, tuberculosis and pneumonia;
- Get emotional support by seeking counselling and joining support groups;
- Learn how to manage HIV related stress.

2.3.3. Modalities of VCT

VCT has continued to expand with the number of facilities globally offering the services. To increase and promote awareness of one's HIV status, different models of HIV delivery have been developed to reach individuals, couples and families not only through different clinic settings and provider initiated settings, but also by bringing VCT closer to people in their families and communities through mobile and home-based testing approaches (Labhart, Motlomelo, Cerutti, Pfeiffer, Kamele, Hobbins & Ehmer, 2014; Fonner, Denison, Kennedy, O'Reilly & Sweat, 2012).

- Flynn, Johnson, Sands et al., (2017) report that only 42% of countries permit lay providers to perform HIV testing and 50% are allowed to administer pre and post-test counselling. The authors thus, propose that due to low uptake of provider use globally and their proven use in increasing HIV testing, countries should consider revising policies to support lay providers using rapid diagnostic tests.
- Research by Kennedy, Yeh, Johnson and Baggaley (2017), propose that new strategies to achieve the UN 90-90-90 targets, health worker shortages, task sharing with trained lay providers is needed
- Labhart et al. (2014) reveal from their study titled "Home-based versus Mobile clinic HIV testing and counselling in rural Lesotho: A cluster randomized trial" that, HIV testing and counselling (HTC) uptake was higher in the home-based than in the mobile clinic group. More first time testers, mainly among adolescents and young adults and a higher proportion of men among participants were reached.

2.3.4. Challenges of Providing Quality VCT for Youth

- Lack of education about VCT among youth;
- Low motivation or reluctance to use VCT services for fear of stigma and discrimination that people who test seropositive may face;
- Ethical considerations such as the need to protect them from discrimination;
- Lack of service availability in resource poor settings;
- Lack of youth friendly services (UNICEF, 2012).

2.3.5. Overcoming Barriers Related to Expansion of VCT Services

Overcoming challenges related to VCT services could motivate more people to inquire about their HIV status.

- Improving the effectiveness of VCT by using efficient HIV testing methods and strategies.
- Improving information and communication to advocate the benefits of VCT and raising community awareness.
- Integrating VCT into other health and social services may also improve access and effectiveness as well as reducing costs.
- Publicizing the benefits of VCT such as sexual behavioural change and opportunity to prevent mother-to-child transmission of HIV.
- Understanding the needs of vulnerable groups. Community participation and involvement of PLWHA is essential for the services to be acceptable and relevant.

2.3.6. Conclusion

VCT is an important component of HIV prevention programme and a critical entry point into HIV care and treatment. As a prevention strategy VCT can influence behaviour change through individual counselling, acquisition of HIV/AIDS knowledge and awareness about one's status. Various innovative and effective interventions for HIV prevention can succeed if more people become aware of their HIV status.

2.4. Vaginal Microbicides

In view of the HIV pandemic, different prophylactic methods including vaginal microbicide preparations are being encouraged as ways to reduce the infection. Without a preventive HIV vaccine, microbicides offer an alternative to condoms as the most feasible method for primary prevention for HIV. Vaginal microbicides can provide a woman-initiated prevention strategy that will substantially reduce the rates of HIV infection.

The availability of microbicides would greatly empower women to protect themselves and their partners. As compared to male or female condoms, vaginal microbicides are a potential preventative option that women can easily control and do not require the cooperation, consent or even knowledge of the partner (WHO, 2007).

2.4.1. Definition

Vaginal microbicides are topical, self-administered products that are designed for application at vaginal or mucosae to inhibit or block early events in HIV infection and thereby prevent transmission of HIV (Ferguson & Rohan, 2011). The WHO (2007) define microbicides as compounds that can be applied inside the vagina or rectum to protect against STIs including HIV. They can be formulated as gels, creams, films, or suppositories. Microbicides may or may not have spermicidal activity.

2.4.2. How Microbicides Function

Microbicides act differently to prevent infection with genital pathogens:

- Some microbicides (Carraguard, Cyanoviran, cellulose sulphate, PRO 2000) provide a physical barrier that keeps HIV and other pathogens from reaching the target cells.
- Another class of microbicides (Acidform, Buffer Gel, & Lactobacillus crispatus) act by enhancing the natural vaginal defence mechanisms and maintaining an acid pH, which protects the vagina.
- Products such as tenoforvir, acts by preventing replication of the virus after it has entered the cell

2.4.3. Development of microbicides

The earliest microbicides candidates developed have been formulated as coitally dependent gels and creams. All microbicides candidates tested in Phase 3 clinical trials so far, have been gel products with non-specific mechanisms of action.

- Recently, research is focussing on compounds containing highly potential and specific ARVs being formulated as primary dosage forms such as vaginal gels or in alternative dosage forms namely, fast dissolve films and tablets.
- Development of combination products of highly active antiviral drugs such as reverse transcriptase inhibitors and entry inhibitors that would be more effective and would reduce the possibility of drug resistance (Garg et al., 2010).

Several studies conducted on the efficacy of microbicides point to the acceptability of these products indicating that they could play a significant role in reducing HIV infection:

- Joanis and Hart (2010) conducted a study on the acceptability of a non-woven device for vaginal drug delivery of microbicides or other active agents. Women found the concept of using a non-woven textile material for vaginal drug delivery acceptable for use in delivering yeast medications and STI/HIV preventatives.
- A study of Muslim women's reflections on the acceptability of vaginal microbicide products to prevent HIV infection, revealed the effectiveness of a microbicide preparation in reducing the risk of HIV infection and the acceptability of microbicide products being linked to a variety of religious persuations and ideals (Hoel, Shaikh & Kagee, 2011).
- According to Ferguson and Rohan (2011), significant protection of women by vaginally applied teneforvir gel in the CAPRISA 004 trial has proven that microbicides can be effective.

2.4.4. Conclusion

The increased incidence of HIV/AIDS disease amongst youth and women has identified an urgent need for a woman controlled efficacious and safe vaginal topical microbicide. Non-ARV microbicides were previously explored as a method of preventing sexual transmission of HIV infection. With the challenges experienced in pursuing this process, there was a shift in focus to develop microbicides containing small molecules of antiviral drugs.

3. BEHAVIOURAL INTERVENTION

Behavioural intervention aims to reduce risk for HIV by promoting condom use and preventing risky sexual behaviours among young people.

3.1. Condom Use among Youth

3.1.1. Introduction

The condom is hailed as the most popularly used contraceptive method among young people. Condoms have been well studied in laboratory tests and it has been determined that they are impermeable to HIV. They are physical barriers that can reduce the risk of a sexual exposure to HIV because they are made of materials that do not allow HIV to pass through them. This makes condoms a highly effective strategy to reduce the risk of HIV transmission when used consistently and/or correctly. They can also provide protection from unplanned pregnancies and other STI's.

3.1.2. Types of Condoms Available to Prevent HIV Transmission
Types of condoms include:

- The *external condom also known as the male condom,* is a sheath made from polyurethane latex or poly-soprene which covers the penis during sexual intercourse. The internal condom, female condom is a pouch made of polyurethane or nitrite. Male condoms have been used for more than 400 years and their female counterparts have been available since 1980.

- The *internal condom* or *female condom* is designed for vaginal but can also be used for anal sex. The pouch is open at one end and closed at the other, with a flexible ring at both ends. The ring at the closed end is inserted into the vagina or anus to hold the condom in place. The ring at the open end of the pouch remains outside of the vagina or anus. Despite their effectiveness, research indicates that condoms are often not used consistently and correctly.

3.1.3. Using Condoms Correctly and Consistently

It is important to use condoms correctly and consistently when engaging in sexual intercourse if they have to serve their purpose effectively. Incorrect use of condoms can cause breakage, slip or leak which can compromise their effectiveness by allowing vulnerable body parts to come in contact with fluids containing HIV. Incorrect use of condoms, such as putting it on too late or removing too early when having sex can increase the risk of HIV transmission (Hendrikson, Pettifor, Sung-Jae, Coates and Rees 2006: Maja, Ehlers, Lewis et al., 2018). Appropriate use of condoms entail:

- Using the correct size, not too big nor too tight.
- Storing condoms at room temperature and regularly replacing those kept in a purse or pocket.
- Checking and discarding expired condoms.
- Ensuring that packaging is not damaged and carefully opening pack without using sharp instruments;
- Using a new condom for every act of vaginal or anal sex;
- Using new condom with every partner and when sharing sex toys;
- Using condoms from start to end;
- Putting on and taking it off correcting.
- Crosby, Yarber, Graham and Sanders (2010) reveal from their study entitled 'Does it fit okay? Problems with condom use as a function of Self-Reported Poor fit', that ill-fitting condoms could easily break, slip, interfere with erection and delay orgasm.

- Common errors, not using condoms throughout sexual intercourse, not leaving space at the tip, not squeezing air from the tip, incorrect withdrawal of condom and condom-associated erection problems were reportedly problems of inconsistent use of condoms (Sanders, Yarber, Kaufman, Crosby, Graham & Milhausen, 2012).
- A study to determine predictors of condom use during participant's recent sexual intercourse, Hendrikson et al., (2006) showed that condom use at sexual debut and talking to one's first sexual partner about condoms were the most significant predictors of condom use at most recent intercourse. Other significant predictors included high condom use, self-efficacy, optimism about the future and behaviour change attributable to HIV/AIDS.
- Mulumeoderhwa (2018) report that most students identified condoms as unsafe and untrustworthy. Reasons given were: condoms do not prevent STIs, HIV and pregnancies, they encourage inappropriate sexual activity and that students preferred flesh-to-flesh sex rather than condoms although few participants acknowledged the importance of condoms. Despite the risk of HIV transmission, boys believe that it is appropriate to have concurrent sexual partnerships.
- The CDC's 2014 School Health Policies and Practice Study found that in the US high schools, education about proper condom use was limited and that only 35% of students were taught how to use them; 55% were informed about the importance of using the dual method to prevent STI's and HIV infection including unplanned pregnancies; 50% of high school progammes taught students how to obtain condoms and only 7% of high schools made condoms available for students at school.
- The CDC's 2015 Youth Risk Behaviour Survey indicate that 43% of sexually active US high school students failed to use condoms during their last sexual encounter.
- The South African Household Survey on HIV Report by the Human Sciences Research Council (HSRC) point out that most adolescents initiate sexual activity early with multiple partners and

inconsistently use condoms. Estimates were that 67% of young people aged 15-24 years reported using condoms at their last sexual encounter down from 85,2% in 2008. Among 25-49 years, condom use fell from 44.1% to 36.1% over the same period. Condom use was reported to be low among clinic attendees in high HIV prevalence settings of Kwa-Zulu Natal despite being informed about the benefits of using condoms consistently (HSRC, 2012).

3.1.4. Barriers of Condom Use amongst Youth

Various barriers can impact negatively on effective use of condoms:

- Cost of condoms for the unemployed youth;
- Moral values;
- Ethnic and religious factors;
- Gender inequality;
- Lack of dialogue between partners;
- Stigma;
- Consumption of alcohol or use of drugs prior to sexual intercourse;
- Anxiety and depression;
- Discomfort due to tightly fitting condoms;
- Breakages;
- Personal aversion to the condom (Mulumeoderhwa, 2018; Sankar, 2008)

Health care providers are therefore urged to:

- Provide comprehensive sexual health education to youth;
- Increase belief in condom effectiveness in preventing HIV infection;
- Increase ability to communicate with partners about STI's and HIV;
- Reinforce the perception that condom use is a norm among peers;

- Develop skills to discuss condom use with doctors.

3.1.5. Conclusion

Condoms remain an essential component of the HIV response. Supporting condom access and use provides effective HIV prevention for millions of people. Condoms allow young people to protect themselves from other STIs including unintended pregnancies.

3.2. Sexual Behaviour of Youth and HIV/AIDS

3.2.1. Introduction

Young people aged 10-24 years and adolescents 10-19 years, especially women, continue to be disproportionately affected by STIs, HIV and unplanned pregnancies as a result of engaging in risky sexual behaviours (Doyle, Mavedzenge and Plummer 2012; Shisana, Rehle, Simbayi et al. 2002.). The South African National Youth Risk Behaviour Survey (2017), report that 21% of all new HIV diagnoses were among young people aged 13-24 years in 2017. Young girls have up to eight times more infection than their male peers. This vulnerability is compounded by structural, social and biological factors which include: exclusion from economic opportunities; lack of access to schooling; experience of gender-based violence and disempowerment of women.

3.2.2. Sexuality and Sexual Identity

Many individuals begin to start exploring their sexuality and sexual identity during adolescence. This implies dating, having sexual intercourse or even marriage. Cultural norms, stigmas and taboos related to sexual debut and sexual activity during adolescence vary between countries. Age of first sex or sexual debut varies across countries and regions but is impacted by cultural and religious norms around early marriage as well as prevalence of experiences of sexual violence. Research conducted among school children in eight African countries (Peltzer, 2010), indicate that 27.3% respondents had their sexual debut before age 15 years, 38.1% boys and 15.8% were girls. Factors associated with early sexual debut were identified as: not living with both biological parents; lack of parental monitoring and connectedness; having more advanced physical maturity; having more permissive attitudes towards sex; alcohol abuse; school problems and depressive symptoms for girls.

Peltzer and Pengpid (2015) mention that a quarter of the sample in their study of six Caribbean countries, (26.9%) had experienced sexual debut before the age of 15 years, 37.2% among boys and 16.9% were girls. In multivariate logistic regression analysis, male gender, substance abuse, truancy and lack of parents or guardian attachment were associated with early sexual debut.

Many sexually vulnerable young people such as women, self-identifying gay men and transgender youth in low-resource settings may be more likely to engage in cross-generational and transactional sex relationships as well as formal sex work. Adolescents in conflict or refugee settings may also have even less control on their sexual experience due to the chaos of their surroundings, and may exchange sex for food, housing or health services.

Male adolescents across the globe are more likely to engage in sexual activity and at an earlier age than their female counterparts (Bearinger et al., 2006, cited by Moukhyer, Kaplan, Lazarevich, Salinas, Kahn, Maja & Julie, 2018). This is likely due to males feeling the need to prove their "virility" and social taboos against girls being sexually active and sexual beings.

Furthermore, many young girls who are sexually active engage in sexual relations with multiple partners which have major public health implications for transmission of STIs and HIV infection.

3.2.3. Gender Identity and Sexual Orientation

As sexual feelings begin to develop, adolescents may find themselves more attracted to the opposite sex, the same sex or both sexes. Additionally, they may feel that they identify with being a man, woman or gender non-conforming, regardless of their natal gender. Across the globe, adolescents struggle with understanding what their gender and sexual identities are and to whom they are attracted. In many cultures it is believed that anatomy should dictate gender, and opposite genders should attract. In some cultures, gender is viewed in binary terms- male/female, man/woman, whereas in other cultures, there may be three or more genders and/or gender may be viewed more along a spectrum. In reality, individuals are different and their feelings and desires may not follow social norms.

Perhaps because of the lack of binding treaties, but more likely due to deeply entrenched cultural and religious norms, adolescents are persecuted all over the world for "living their sexual orientation". Sexuality is a topic which is particularly sensitive, and infractions on human rights can be justified through cultural sovereignty or "traditional values" (Moukyer et al., 2018). While the topic should be approached delicately in some more conservative countries, lesbians, gay and gender non-conforming youth are often abused and are at higher risk to contract STIs/HIV. To cope with structural discrimination and stigma, they may be more likely to engage in other high-risk behaviours such as alcohol and substance use. As a health care provider, it is important to make adolescents of all sexual orientations and gender identities feel comfortable discussing their health concerns and issues without judgement to be able to provide appropriate healthcare for their specific needs.

3.2.4. Substance Abuse and Alcohol Consumption

Substance and alcohol abuse contribute to HIV transmission by increasing the risk of unsafe sex among both HIV positive and HIV negative populations. Illicit drug use occurs at high rates among HIV positive individuals and has health consequences for users. Long term drug abuse can interfere with normal brain activity and metabolism as well as becoming a chronic relapsing condition. The use of drugs and excessive alcohol by HIV infected individuals decreases their likelihood of using ART, adhering to treatment and achieving effective viral suppression (Burman et al., 2001). Davis, Masters, Eakins, Danube, George, Morris and Herman (2014) assert that alcohol intoxication directly decreased women's intentions to use condoms in the future

3.2.5. Conclusion

Adolescents and youth continue to be vulnerable to risky sexual behaviours which often result in unintended pregnancies and STIs including HIV/AIDS. Addressing these challenges is critical given the rising numbers of new HIV infections among young people.

4. STRUCTURAL INTERVENTION

Structural intervention in this section, incorporates stigma, discrimination including promotion of youth friendly services.

4.1. HIV Related Stigma and Discrimination

4.1.1. Introduction

HIV-related stigma and discrimination are major barriers to the successful control of HIV infection. HIV-related stigma entails negative beliefs, feelings and attitudes towards PLWHA, their families, HIV service providers, members of groups that have been heavily impacted by HIV.

Link and Phelan (2001) describe stigma as a harmful societal phenomenon, enabled by underlying social, political and economic powers that begins when a difference is labelled and linked to negative stereotypes leading to a separation of "us" from "them" and finally of status loss and discrimination for those carrying the trait.

HIV related discrimination refers to the unfair and unjust treatment of someone based on the real or perceived HIV status. Discrimination also affect families or friends and those who care for PLWHA. HIV discrimination is also fuelled by myths of casual transmission of HIV and pre-existing biases against certain groups, certain sexual behaviours, drug use and fear of illness practices (Karamouzin, Maryam, Ali-Akbar & Zolala, 2015; Senyolo, Maja & Ramukumba, 2015).

These include gay and bisexual men, homeless people, street youth and mentally ill people. Discrimination can be institutionalised through laws, policies and

Deacon (2006) suggest that HIV related discrimination be analysed separately from stigma to explore the range of stigma related disadvantages that may result from the stigmatization process and positive responses such as resilience and activism.

4.1.2. Domains of the Stigmatization Process

Domains of the stigmatization process include drivers, facilitators, intersecting stigmas and manifestations of stigma.

Drivers are individual-level factors that negatively influence the stigmatization process such as lack of awareness of stigma and its harmful consequences, fear of HIV infection through casual contact with PLWHA, fear of economic ramifications or social breakdown due to HIV positive family and community members and prejudice and stereotypes towards PLWHA and key populations at higher risk of HIV infection.

Karamouzin et al., (2015) report types of stigma as: internal stigma (silence, shame and feeling miserable) and external stigma (from their families, communities and health care providers).

Furthermore, Chirowodza, Ntogwisangu, Srivak, Modiba, Murima and Fritz (2009) indicate fear that contributes to HIV stigma and discrimination as fear of transmission, fear of suffering and death and the burden of caring for PLWHA

Facilitators are societal level factors that influence the stigmatization process either negatively or positively including protective or punitive laws, availability of grievance redress systems, awareness of rights, structural barriers at public policy level, cultural and gender norms, existence of social support for PLWHA and powerlessness among PLWHA to resist and overcome the manifestations of stigma.

Intersecting or layered stigmas refer to the multiple stigmas that people often face due to HIV status, gender, profession, migrants, drug use, poverty, marital status, sexual and gender orientation.

4.1.3. Intervention Strategies for Stigma and Discrimination against PLWHA

HIV/AIDS related stigma and discrimination are barriers to HIV prevention, effectiveness, VCT uptake and accessing care in many clinical settings. Efforts to address stigma and discrimination could be enforced in the following ways:

- *Information-based approaches* such as information in brochures, print media, radio and drama. Young people often lack knowledge regarding sexuality issues and have misconceptions about contraceptives and their side effects. They need to be provided with accurate information and given opportunities to ask questions and discuss their concerns. Mass media (radio and television programmes), peer education and intra-personal communication have been used successfully to communicate health information to young people and influence their norms (Odimegwu, Alabi, De Wet & Akinyemi, 2018).
- *Life skills building* which includes participatory learning sessions to reduce negative attitudes. Life skills enhance the quality of life and prevent dysfunctional behaviours.

  The Association of African Universities (2004) and HEADS (2010) highlight that programmes offered at tertiary education institutions should consider the socio-economic factors affecting students' quality of life and their vulnerability to HIV and AIDS. Most universities have integrated HIV and AIDS into their curricula to equip learners with better skills to prevent risky sexual behaviours.

  The South African Departments of Health and Education embarked on a national programme to implement life skills training, sexuality and AIDS education in secondary schools since 1995 to increase knowledge and skills needed for healthy relationships, effective community and responsible decision-making that would protect learners from HIV infection (Department of Education, 1997/8; Department of Health, 1997/8).

- *Counselling for PLWHA.*

    Counselling for risk reduction in HIV prevention deals with medical, psychosocial and social issues. The risk reduction approach for adolescents and youth includes exploring their feelings about sexual activity, using their existing HIV knowledge as an engaging tool, addressing the barriers they have for safer sex, focusing on perceptions that might affect risky behaviour and referral. Some HIV care providers use motivational interviewing for guidance in considering the client's readiness to change their risky behaviour (Kanekar, 2011; Rutledge, 2007).

- *Support groups PLWHA and the general public.*

    The stigma surrounding PLWHA makes life difficult for them and their families. PLWHA often experience, loneliness, stress, depression, guilt, anxiety and loss of self-esteem. They need emotional, spiritual, psycho-social, physical and clinical support to cope better with the condition. Different people and institutions provide such support although it's important for PLWHA to come together, support each other and share their lived experiences of living with HIV/AIDS. Their common needs include:

    - Health and medical services;
    - Counselling to reduce isolation and promote acceptance;
    - Community support groups to provide a safe place where feelings and advice can be shared;
    - Spiritual support such as prayer groups and home visits by religious leaders;
    - Social acceptance to help PLWHA feel welcome by visiting them and treating them like friends;
    - Physical care which includes bathing, cleaning when sick;
    - Nutritional help using affordable and available food;
    - Safe clean water either boiled or treated with chlorine;
    - Accurate information about HIV/AIDS.

4.1.4. Conclusion

HIV/AIDS-related stigma poses a problem for all in communities thereby imposing severe hardships on the people who are targets, ultimately interfering with treatment. Emphasis on the eradication of AIDS related stigma would assist in creating a social climate conducive to a compassionate response to this epidemic. Eliminating all forms of HIV/AIDS related stigma and discrimination is fundamental in achieving the Sustainable Developmental Goals and targets by 2030 including ending HIV/AIDS.

4.2. Adolescent/Youth Friendly Health Services

4.2.1. Introduction

Young people are often not considered in National HIV and AIDS plans which typically focus on adults and children. As a result, there is lack of or limited adolescent/youth friendly health services. Adolescent/Youth-Friendly Health Services (A/YFHS) is the gold standard for providing adolescents health services, but implementation of Y/AFHS is often non-existent or has varying quality (Chandra-Mouli et al., 2015). Reproductive Health Services in consultation with the WHO (2012) recommend the following for adolescent/youth friendly services:

- A/YFS with the adoption of 'life-cycle approach' to HIV prevention which responds to the changing contexts that people face at different ages.
- Age-appropriate services. Young people respond much better to HIV and SRHR services that are specific to their age group. Targeted counselling to encourage behaviour change among young people is more effective than just handing out condoms.
- Engaging parents, care givers and guardians in the response. Stakeholders such as parents, health care providers and community leaders are key to HIV prevention.

- Engaging schools as they have the potential to provide detailed education on HIV and AIDS including other SRHR issues.
- Engaging young people because they have the potential to be great peer educators and to help in the design of HIV related services and programmes. Technology and social media play an important role to engage young people in sharing HIV knowledge.
- Transition to adulthood. Consideration that young people will have less support from their families and communities as they transition working and living independently.

Evaluations have shown that adolescent's use of SRH services can be increased when the following complementary approaches are implemented together (Chandra-Mouli et al., 2015: Moukyer et al. 2019).

- Providers are trained and supported to be nonjudgmental and friendly to adolescent/youth clients.
- Health facilities are welcoming and appealing.
- Management System, policies and processes support the effective provision of youth/adolescent services.
- Communication and outreach activities inform adolescents/youth about services and encourage them to make use of services.
- Provision of relevant information, education and communicating promotion behaviour change.
- Community members are supportive of the importance of providing health services to adolescents and youth.

4.3. Conclusion

Young people are unwilling to visit health facilities for contraceptives and other health services because they view them as unfriendly. To be considered adolescent/youth friendly, health services should be accessible, acceptable, equitable, appropriate and effective to adolescents and youth.

5. Innovative Use of Technology for Prevention of HIV

5.1. Introduction

Perhaps the most effective and prompt strategy of addressing HIV and AIDS is the innovative use of technology. This section outlines various technological ways of communicating and sharing information from individual to groups, from far and near and from developed to underdeveloped communities.

Popular mobile technologies are described as belonging to one or more of the following categories: Cell phones, social media, computers/internet as well as native and cloud based applications (Swendeman & Rotheram-Borus, 2010; Cornelius et al., 2013; Young & Chiu, 2014).

5.1.1. Cell Phones

Cell phones facilitate multiple forms of communication such as phone calls, text messages and multimedia messaging services which include video and picture texts. In most countries, youth between ages 18-29, communicate with each other predominantly through text messaging. Recent HIV interventions targeting youth have utilised text messages to reduce substance abuse and increase HIV counselling and testing (Reebak et al., 2012; Cornelius et al., 2013). The use of cell phones in health care is often referred to as mHealth, one of the fastest growing technology in medicine in developing countries.

- In Uganda, 64% of 176 HIV infected patients with access to cell phones received reminders via voice calls or text messages about missed clinic appointments. Almost 80% of those who had missed their appointments and were contacted via cell phone, came in for their first visit within two days of the contact (Kunutsor, Walley, Katabira et al., 2010).

- A randomized study was conducted in Kenya and participants received daily or weekly texts to improve adherence. The outcome was that 53% respondents achieved adherence rates of 90% during the 48week study compared to 40% of the control group.
- In developed countries such as Australia, adolescents who received text messages about STDs, demonstrated increased knowledge about STDs and had fewer sexual partners compared to a group that received messages about sun safety.
- In the United States of America, researchers had sent HIV prevention text messages stressing the importance of condom use and reducing the number of sexual partners. Those who received messages were more likely to become monogamous than the control group (Wright, Fortune, Juzang et al., 2011).

5.2. Social Media

Social media is computer-based and cell phone technology that facilitates the sharing of ideas, thoughts and information through the building of virtual networks and communication. It is internet-based and gives users quick electronic communication of content. Social media can have a tremendous impact on HIV research because these technologies can serve as platforms and services that enable individuals to engage in communication from one-to-one, one-to-many and many-to-many (Taggart, Grewe, Conserve, Gliwa & Isler, 2015; Nguyen, Gold, Pedrana, Chang, Howard, et al., 2013).

5.2.1. Types of Social Media

Different patterns of social media exist based on socio-economic, regional and language factors. Before incorporating these technologies, researchers should understand the trends and how they impact on HIV risk. Types of social media commonly used:

- Social Networks such as Facebook, WhatsApp, Instagram, Linked in, Twitter;
- Bookmarking sites, which include Pinterest, Flipboard and Digg;
- Social News, such as Digg;
- Media sharing, for example, Pinterest, You Tube;
- Microblogging, for example, Twitter, Facebook;
- Blog comments and forums;
- Social Review sites;
- Community Bloggs.

5.3. Computers and Internet

Computers and internets are vehicles for providing promising interventions in addressing various forms of health related problems including HIV/AIDS. The privacy offered by computers and internet is significant as it's accessibility to interventions from multiple sites. The standardization, fidelity, ease of replication of computer-based interventions and the added potential benefits of reach and increased use of internet by youth make both computers and internet logical venues for HIV/STD research and prevention interventions. The Internet has been used effectively to increase access to care among PLWHA and patients with eating disorders. Internet offers an additional opportunity to reach larger numbers of people in diverse settings.

Studies demonstrating the efficacy of computer-based interventions for HIV and STD prevention, delivered via computers in various institutional and community settings highlight the following:

- Kiene and colleagues showed that college students randomized to participate in two computer-based sessions to reduce HIV and STD risk spaced two weeks apart, had an increase in awareness regarding HIV and STD, more frequently carried and used

condoms often compared to the control group (Kiene & Barta, 2006).
- Lightfoot and colleagues report that high-risk youth participating in two five-hour computer-based HIV intervention sessions were less likely to engage in sex and had fewer sex partners compared to control groups (Lightfoot, Comulada & Stover, 2007).

5.4. Advantages of Using Computer-based technology

- Cost of implementing computers is minimal compared with those requiring significant human resources;
- Intervention fidelity is maintained through the standardization of content by use of computer algorithms;
- Includes features such as interactivity and multimedia which may aid in the fostering of behavioural change and computerized interventions;
- people to internet;
- Increases productivity;
- Can store vast amounts of information and reduce waste;
- Helps sort, organize and search through information;
- Helps people to learn and be informed

5.5. Cloud-Native Based Applications

Cloud-Native technology is an approach to building applications and services specifically for a cloud environment. They are used to develop applications built with services packaged in containers, deployed as micro services and managed on elastic infrastructure through agile DevOps processes and continuous delivery workflows (Craven, 2019). It is an approach to building and running applications that exploits the advantages of the cloud computing delivery model. Mostly, it has the ability to offer nearly limitless computer power, on-demand along with data and application services for its developers.

DevOps is the collaboration between software developers and IT operators with the goal of constantly delivering high quality software that solves customer challenges. It has the potential to create a culture and an environment where building, testing and releasing software happens rapidly and more consistently. With the cloud, users can access applications through an internet connection

5.6. Conclusion

Technology is advancing rapidly and becoming a cost effective trend in communication, sharing information among young people and adults. Information shared can be educational, health promotion, politics, social and for research purposes. Mobile cell phones are being used for communicating on one to one basis, amongst small and large groups to share information by calls, text-messaging, videos, pictures to people from far and around. Social media operating via cell phone, computers and internet is expanding with the latest developments sharing with peers, colleagues, families and communities. These technology-based tools hold much promise to offer better interventions in eradicating HIV/AIDS, thereby achieving the Sustainable Development Goals by 2030.

REFERENCES

Bukenya, D, Mayanja, BN, Nakamanya, S, Muhumuza, R & Seeley, J. 2019. What causes non-adherence among some individuals on long-term antiretroviral therapy? Experiences of individuals with poor viral suppression in Uganda. *AIDS Research and Therapy,* 16(2).

Chandra-Mouli, V, McCarraher, DR, Phillips, SJ, Williamson, N & Hainsworth, G. 2014. Contraception for adolescents in low and middle income countries: needs, barriers and access. 2014. *Reproductive Health*, 11(1).

Cornelius, J, Kennedy, A. & Wesslan, R. 2019. An Examination of Twitter data to identify Risky Sexual Practices Among Youth and Young adults in Botswana. International. *Journal of Environmental Research and Public Health*, 16(4): 656.

Cornelius, JB, Dmochowski, J, Boyer, C, St Lawrence, J, Lightfoot, M & Moore, M. 2013. Text Messaging Enhanced HIV Intervention for African American Adolescents. A feasibility Study. *Journal of the Association of Nurses in AIDS care*, 24(3): 256-267.

Cutler, B & Justman, J. 2008. Vaginal microbicides and Prevention of HIV transmission. *Lancet; Infectious Diseases*, 8(11): 685-697.

Davis, KC, Masters, NT, Eakins, D, Danube, L, George, WH, Morris, J & Heiman, JR. 2014. Alcohol Intoxication and Condom Use Self-Efficacy Effects on Women's Condom Use Intentions. *Addict. Behaviour*, 39(1): 153-158.

Deacon, H. 2006. Towards a sustainable theory of health related stigma: Lessons from the HIV/AIDS literature. *Community Appl. Soc. Psych*, (16): 418-425.

Den Brinker, M, Wit, FW, Wertheim-van Dillen, PM et al. 2000. Hepatitis B and C virus co-infection and the risk of hepatotoxicity of highly active ARV in HIV-1 infection. *AIDS,* 14(18):2895-2902.

Doyle, AM, Mavedzenge, SN, Plummer, Ross, D. 2012. The Sexual Behaviour of adolescents in sub Saharan Africa: Patterns and Trends from National Surveys. *European Journal of Tropical Medicine and International Health*, 17(7): 796-807.

Doggett, E, Lanham, M, Wilcher, R, Gafos, M, Karim, QA, & Heise, L. 2015. Optimizing HIV Prevention for Women: A Review of Evidence From Microbicide Studies and Considerations for Gender-Sensitive microbicides. *International AIDS Society*, 18(1): 20536.

Duggan, M. 2013. *Cell phone Activities.* PEW Research Centre.

Dunkle, KL & Jewkes, R. 2007. Effective HIV prevention requires gender transformative work with men. *Sexually transmitted Infections*, 83(3)): 173-174.

Ferguson, LM, & Rohan, LC. 2011. The importance of the Vaginal Delivery Route for ARVs in HIV Prevention. *Ther Deliv*, 2(12): 535-550.

Fonner, VA, Denison, J, Kennedy, C, O'reilly, K, & Swart, M. 2012. *VCT for changing HIV- related risk behaviour in developing countries: Cochrane Database System Rev*, 12:9:CD001224.

Flynn, DE, Johnson, C, Sands, A, Wong, V, Figueroa, C & Baggaley, R. 2017' Can trained lay Providers Perform HIV Testing Services? A review of National HIV Testing Policies. *BMC Research Notes*, 10(1), 20.

Friend, DR, Clark, JT, Kiser, PF & Clark, MR. 2013. Multipurpose Prevention Technological Products in development, *Antiviral Research*, 100 Supplementary, 539-547.

Garg, S, Goldman, D, Krumme, M, Rohan, LC, Smoot, S & Friend, D. 2010. Advances in Development, Scale-Up and Manufacturing of Microbicide gels, Films and Tablets. *Antiviral Research*, 88, Supplement, 519-529.

Gordon, D. 2013. The Mobile Phone: Effective New Weapon in HIV Prevention. *Patient Care*.

Karamouzian, M, Maryam, A, Ali-Akbar, HS & Zolala, F. 2015. "I am Dead to Them": HIV-related Stigma Experienced by People living with HIV in Kerman, Iran. 2015. *Journal of the Association of Nurses in AIDS Care*, 26(1):46-56.

Karen, R, Barth, MD, Robert, L, Cook, MD, Downs, SJ, Galen, ES & Fischoff, B. 2002. Social Stigma and Negative Consequences: Factors that influence College students' decision to seek testing for Sexually transmitted infections. *Journal of American College Health*, 50(4):153-159.

Kelly, CG & Shatlock, RJ. 2011. Specific microbicides in the Prevention of HIV infection. *International Medicine*, 270(6): 509-519.

Kennedy, CE, Yeh, PT, Johnson, C & Baggaley, R. 2017. Should trained lay providers perform HIV testing? A Systematic review to inform the WHO guidelines. *AIDS Care*, 29(12):1473-1479.

Kepe, T. 2010. Secrts that kill: Crisis, custodianship and responsibilities in ritual male circumcision in the Eastern Cape Province. *South African Social Sciences and Medicine*, 70(5):729-735.

Kiene, SM & Barta, WD. 2006. A brief individualised Computer-delivered sexual risk reduction intervention increases HIV AIDS prevention behaviour. *Journal of Adolescent Health,* 39: 404-410.

Labhart, ND, Motlomelo, M, Cerutti, B, Pfeiffer, K, Kamele, M, Hobbins, MA & Ehmer, J. 2014. Home-based versus Mobile clinic HIV Testing and Counselling in rural Lesotho: A Cluster Randomized Trial. 2014. PLoS Med, 11(12) e1001768.

Lightfoot, M, Comulada, WS, & Stover, G.2007. Computerized HIV prevention intervention for adolescents: indicators for efficacy. *American Journal of Public Health,* 97:1027-1030.

Link, B & Phelan, J. 2001. Conceptualizing Stigma. *Annual Research and Social,* (27): 363-385.

Maja, TMM, Ehlers, VJ, Lewis, J, Bistany, GC & Alimena, S. 2018. Contraception: An Educational Resource for Health Professions Students. *Women and Health Together For the Future, Global Health for Education Training and Service.* USA./Cape Town, SA.

Mallal, S, Phillips, E, Carosi, et al. 2008. HLA-*B5701 Screening for hypersensitivity to abacavir. *England Journal of Medicine*, 358(6): 568-579.

Marston, M, Beguy, D, Kabiru, C & Cleland, J. 2013. *Predictors of Sexual debut among young adolescents in Nairobi's informal settlements.*

Moukyer, M, Kaplan, KC, Lazarevich, I, Salinas, AA, Kahn, M, Maja, TM & Julie, H. 2018. *Adolescent Health: Women and Health Learning Package: An Educational Resource.* GHETS, USA/Cape Town, SA.

Mulumeoderhwa, M. 2018. It's not good to eat a Candy in a Wrapper: Male students' Perspectives on Condom Use and concurrent Sexual Partnerships in the Eastern Democratic Republic of Congo. *SAHARA Journal*, 15(1):89-102.

National Department of Health. *National Strategic Plan on HIV, STIs and TB: 2012-2016.*

Nguyen, P, Gold, J, Pediana, A, Chang, S, Howard, S, Ilic, O, Hollard, M & Stoove, M. 2013. Sexual Health Promotion on Social Networking sites: A Process Evaluation of the Face Space Project. *Adolescence and Health*, 53(1):98-104.

Ntombana, L. 2011. Should Xhosa male initiation be abolished? *Journal of Cultural Studies,* 14(6):631-640.

Noar, S. 2011. Computer technology-based interventions in HIV prevention: State of evidence and future directions. *Psychological and Socio-medical Aspects of HIV/AIDS,* 23:5.

Noar, SM, Black, HG. & Larson, PB. 2009. Efficacy of computer technology-based HIV prevention interventions: a meta-analysis. *Epedimiology and Social,* 23(1):107-115.

Odimegwu, CO, Alabi, O, De Wet, N, & Akinyemi, JO. 2018. Ethnic heterogeneity in the determinants of HIV/AIDS Stigma and Discrimination among Nigerian women. *BMC Public Health,* (18): 763.

Peltzer, K. & Pengpid, S. 2015. Early sexual debut and Adolecsent Factors Among in-school adolescents in six Caribbean countries. *West Indian Medical Journal,* 64(4):35-56.

Peltzer, K. 2010. Early Sexual Debut and Associated Factors Among In-school adolescents in eight African countries. *Acta Paediatr.,* 99(8):1242-1247.

Plotkin, M, Kuver, J, et al. 2011. Voluntary Medical Male circumcision: matching demand and supply with quality and efficacy high volume campaign in Iringa region, Tanzania. *PLoS Med,* 8: e1001131.

Reebak, C, Grant, D, Fletcher, J, Branson, C, Shoptaw, S, Bowers, J et al. 2012. Text-Messaging reduces HIV Risk Behaviours among Methamphetamine-using men who have sex with men. *AIDS and Behaviour,* 16 (7): 1993-2002.

Rutledge, SE. 2007. Single session motivational enhancement support change towards reduction of HIV transmission by HIV positive persons. *Arch Sexual Behaviour,* 36(2):313-319.

Senyolo, RG, Maja, TMM & Ramukumba, TE. 2015. Stigma experienced by people living with Human Immuno-deficiency virus/AIDS. *Africa*

Journal for Physical, Health education, Recreation and Dance, Supplement, 1:94-106.

Shisana, O, Rehle, T, Simbayi, L et al. 2009. *South African National HIV prevalence, HIV incidence, and communication survey: A turning tide among teenagers?* Cape Town: HRSC Press.

Shisana, O, Rehle, T, Simbayi, L et al. 2012. *South African National HIV prevalence, HIV incidence and behaviour survey.* 2012. Cape Town: HSRC Press.

Swendeman, D & Rotheram-Borus. 2010. Innovations in STD and HIV prevention: Internet and mobile phone delivery vehicles for global diffusion. *Current Opinion Psych,* 23(2):139-144.

Taggart, T, Grewe, EM, Conserve, DF, Gliwa, C & Isler, MR. 2015. Social Media and HIV: A Systematic Review of Uses of Social Media in HIV Communication. *Journal of Medical Internet Research,* 17(11):e248.

Tripathi, AK, Shukla, M, Argawal, MJ, Sing, VR, Strivasta, M, & Singh, VK. 2016. Non-adherence to ART Among PLWHA attending two Tertiary hospitals in District of Northern India. *Indian Journal of Community Medicine,* 41(1): 55-61.

Tso, LS, Tang, W, Li, H, Yan, HY & Tucker, JD.2015. Social media interventions to prevent HIV. A review of interventions and methodological considerations. *Current Opinion Psych,* 1(9): 6-10.

UNAIDS. 2015. *Active involvement of young people is key to ending AIDS epidemic by 2030.*

UNAIDS. 2014. *90-90-90: an ambitious treatment target to help end the AIDS epidemic: Joint UN Programme on HIV/AIDS.* Geneva.

UNICEF. 2013. *Lost in Transitions: Current issues faced by adolescents living with HIV in Asia Pacific.*

Vermund, SH. 2014. Massive benefits of ARV therapy in Africa. *Journal of Infectious diseases,* 209 (4): 483-485.

Vermund, SH. 2006. Millions of life-years saved with potent ARV drugs in the US: a celebration with challenges. *Journal of Infectious Diseases,* 194:1-5.

Walensky, RP, Paltiel, AD, Losina, E et al. 2006. The Survival benefits of AIDS treatment in the US. *Journal of Infectious Diseases,* 194"11-19.

WHO. 2013. *Global update on HIV treatment.* Switzerland: Geneva.

WHO. 2012. *Making health services Adolescent Friendly-Developing National Quality Standards for Adolescent Friendly Services.* Switzerland: Geneva.

WHO. 2010. Adherence to longterm therapies: Evidence for Action. Switzerland: Geneva

Wright, E, Fortune, T, Juzang, I, et al. 2011. Text messaging for HIV prevention with young Black men: formative research and campaign development. *AIDS Care,* 23(5): 534-541.

Ybarra, ML, Mwaba, K, Prescott, TL, Roman, NV, Rooi, B & Bull, S. 2014. *Opportunities for technology-based HIV prevention among high school students in Cape Town.*

Young, S & Chiu, J. 2014. Innovative Use of technology for HIV Prevention and Care: Evidence, Challenges and the way forward. *Journal of Mobile Tecnology and Medicine,* 3(15): 1-3.

In: HIV/AIDS
Editor: Ethel K. Hebert

ISBN: 978-1-53617-923-1
© 2020 Nova Science Publishers, Inc.

Chapter 5

HIV TREATMENT AS PREVENTION

*Zanesha Jeter[1] and Olga M. Klibanov [1,]**
[1]Wingate University School of Pharmacy,
Wingate University, Wingate, NC, US

ABSTRACT

Globally, A Treatment as Prevention (TasP) model has been effectively utilized to avoid perinatal transmission of Human Immunodeficiency Virus (HIV). Evidence is sufficient to expand this principle to the general population of patients with HIV diagnosis. In 2016, the World Health Organization (WHO) issued updated recommendations on the treatment and prevention of HIV infections. Recommendations promote the accelerated initiation of antiretroviral therapy (ART) in all patients diagnosed with HIV, regardless of CD4 count. Patients with HIV have been found to have decreased disease progression with early initiation of ART and subsequent HIV-1 RNA suppression. Other studies have found efficacy in ART as a preventative measure, in the sexual transmission of HIV between mixed-status couples. The WHO offers recommendations to promote the success of TasP with ART, including relaxed HIV-1 RNA monitoring parameters for stable patients, discontinuation of highly toxic drugs in initial therapy,

---

* Corresponding Author's Email: o.klibanov@wingate.edu.

and increased availability and affordability of ARVs. This chapter will outline the updated recommendations, guiding healthcare professionals to employ TasP. Supporting evidence and rationale behind the TasP model for HIV will be reviewed. A discussion of the public health measures necessary to promote the success of TasP is also included.

INTRODUCTION

The Progression of HIV Treatment Strategy

Human Immunodeficiency Virus (HIV) is bloodborne pathogen. This virus can be transmitted via sexual, parenteral, and perinatal modes. The HIV virus attacks immune cells to disable the body's defensive systems. HIV-infected individuals cannot produce the antibodies needed to protect the immune system. Infection occurs in multiple stages, sometimes presenting as clinical latency. During asymptomatic periods, the HIV positive individual is infectious, as RNA continues to replicate. In the acute stage of HIV patients may present with generalized symptoms that mirror that of other illnesses. This creates challenges in screening and subsequent diagnosis. The HIV-1 RNA has emerged as a prognostic factor of HIV disease progression. Untreated HIV will progress to acquired immune deficiency syndrome (AIDS), leaving the patient at risk of acquiring opportunistic infections. Probability of progression to AIDS is dependent on adequate maintenance of HIV-1 RNA. It has been found that treatment with three ARVs from two different pharmacological classes will suppress viral replication to undetectable levels [1, 2].

The first ARV drug, zidovudine (AZT), was approved by the FDA in 1987. In 1997, highly active antiretroviral therapy (HAART) became a treatment standard. That same year, the FDA approved the first combination ART tablet, zidovudine/lamivudine (Combivir®). HAART promoted the combination of ARV drugs to achieve adequate suppression. Advancement in screening services in the early 2000s resulted in increased diagnosis. HIV infection declines began to level out and the healthcare system increased efforts into creating ARV combinations to reduce pill burden. The extraordinary advances in the field of HIV therapeutics over the last 3 decades have led to the FDA approval of dozens of antiretroviral drugs, with most patients now taking a low-pill burden regimen on a daily basis, and having an excellent long-term prognosis [3].

Nevertheless, it is estimated that there are still approximately 36 million people infected with HIV around the world, with 1.8 million becoming newly infected every year and 1 million dying annually from HIV-related causes [4]. Today, many efforts are focusing on ways to prevent HIV transmission. One of the newer strategies to accomplish this is using "treatment as prevention", or TasP, also known as "Undetectable = Untransmittable", or "U = U". Recent studies have shown that when ART is used to suppress the HIV-1 RNA to less than 200 copies/mL, HIV is not transmitted to sexual partners [3].

TasP: Data from Landmark Clinical Trials

The HIV Prevention Trials Network (HPTN) 052 trial was conducted in 9 sites, globally, between 2005 and 2015. HIV-serodiscordant couples were randomized into early or delayed ART treatment groups to assess sexual transmission. This trial concluded that HIV-infected patients receiving early ART had a 93% lower risk of genetically linked partner infection, through sexual transmission, than those who had delayed ART. Patients who had achieved stable HIV RNA suppression transmitted no linked infections in their partners. These data suggest the benefits of early ART as a preventative measure in sexual transmission of HIV [5].

The PARTNER-1 and PARTNER-2 studies further evaluated the risk of sexual transmission by HIV-infected individuals with undetectable HIV-1 RNA. In the PARTNER 1 study, 1166 European serodiscordant couples were observed from September 2010 to May 2014 as they had barrierless sexual intercourse. The HIV positive partner maintained HIV-1 RNA suppression, defined as less than 200 copies/mL, through ART.

Table 1. TasP data from clinical trials [5-8]

Study	Intervention	Primary Endpoint	Primary Endpoint Results	Comments
Heterosexual and Homosexual Men and Women				
HPTN 052 Trial [5] *Phase 3, RCT, PAR, MC*	TDF/FTC (n = 1251) Placebo (n = 1248) Early ART: Immediate initiation of ART (n = 886) Delayed ART: Initiated ART after two consecutive CD4+ counts below 250 cells/mm³ or if an AIDS-related illness developed (n = 877)	Occurrence of genetically linked HIV infection in the previously HIV(-) partner	93% reduction of risk of linked partner infection in early ART [HR 0.07 (95% CI, 0.02 to 0.22]. No linked infections when index participant stably suppressed by ART.	Suggested the benefits of early ART and HIV-1 RNA suppression as a preventative measure in sexual transmission of HIV.
PARTNER-1 Trial [6] *P, OB, MC*	Evaluated transmission of HIV between serodifferent couples, where the HIV(+) partner was taking suppressive ART (n=1166 couples)	Occurrence of genetically linked HIV infection in the previously HIV(-) partner	0 phylogenetically-linked HIV transmissions; upper 95% CI, 0.30/100 couple-years of follow-up. Upper 95% CI for condomless anal sex was 0.71/100 couple-years of follow-up.	No HIV transmission in condom less sex when HIV (+) partner has HIV-1 RNA suppression with ART. Applicable to heterosexual and homosexual couples.

Study	Intervention	Primary Endpoint	Primary Endpoint Results	Comments
Men who Have Sex with Men (MSM)				
PARTNER-2 Trial [7] *P, OB, MC*	Evaluated transmission of HIV between serodifferent homosexual couples, where HIV(+) partner taking suppressive ART (n = 972 couples)	Occurrence of genetically linked HIV infection in the previously HIV(-) partner	0 phylogenetically-linked HIV transmissions; upper 95% CI, 0.23/100 couple-years of follow-up.	In MSMs, no HIV transmission in condomless sex when HIV (+) partner has HIV-1 RNA suppression with ART.
Opposites Attract Trial [8] *P, O3, MC, LC*	Collected attitudinal and behavioral information on factors associated with anally transmitted HIV risk. Evaluated transmission of HIV between serodifferent partners when HIV (+) partner had undetectable HIV-1 RNA from ART. (n=343 couples)	Genetically-linked HIV infection in the previously HIV (-) partner	0 phylogenetically-linked HIV transmissions; upper CI limit of 1.59/100 couple-years of follow-up. Relationship of ≤1year: HIV incidence was approximately 6/100 person-years.	No HIV transmission in condomless sex when HIV (+) partner has HIV-1 RNA suppression with ART. Identified homosexual men in the first year of romantic relationships to be at higher risk of transmitting HIV to a partner.

RCT: randomized control trial; MC: multicenter; PAR: parallel; HR: hazard ratio; LC: longitudinal cohort; P: prospective; MSM: men who have sex with men.

Whereas only 38% of participants in the PARTNER-1 study were men who have sex with men (MSMs) couples, PARTNER-2 focused exclusively on sexual transmission between MSMs. PARTNER-2 extended the trial until July of 2017 for 972 MSM couples. Both studies found that there were no phylogenetically linked sexual transmissions of HIV in couples where the HIV-infected partner had undetectable HIV-1 RNA [6, 7].

Opposites Attract, a 2014 observational, prospective, longitudinal, cohort study collected subjective data along with serological results in relation to HIV transmission in MSMs. TasP methods had not been evaluated in a group that engaged predominantly in anal intercourse, a practice that has 10 times the HIV transmission risk as vaginal intercourse. The study found that MSMs in the first year of romantic relationships, were at a higher risk of transmitting HIV to a partner. The authors suggest targeting these men for immediate initiation of ART to reduce this risk [8].

INCORPORATING TASP INTO THE GUIDELINES

Department of Health and Human Services (DHHS)

Recognizing the recent findings on ART initiation, the Department of Health and Human Services has added information on the use of TasP in HIV guidelines. Patients diagnosed with HIV should be initiated on ART immediately. Transmission to a sexual partner will be prevented as long as HIV-1 RNA levels are maintained below 200 copies/mL. The Partners PrEP Study, conducted in East African heterosexual couples, found that phylogenetically linked HIV infections were limited to the first 6 months of consistent ART [9]. Based on these data, it is suggested that HIV positive individuals continue secondary forms of sexual prevention until HIV-1 RNA has been suppressed for at least 6 months [3].

Patients should be counseled to confirm continued HIV-1 RNA suppression with a qualified medical professional on the recommended monitoring frequency. The DHHS guidelines recommend HIV-1 RNA monitoring within 2 to 4 weeks after initiation of ART. Monitoring should be continued every 4 to 8 weeks until suppression is achieved. Monitoring frequency can be relaxed in patients who have sustained HIV-1 RNA suppression. After 2 years of effective ART, HIV-1 RNA can be assessed every 6 months [3].

Undetectable HIV-1 RNA is attainable only if high levels of adherence are met. In many patients on ART HIV-1 RNA remains suppressed after achieving less than 200 copies/mL; however, 10% of patients interrupt viral suppression in the first year of ART due to nonadherence. Studies have shown that HIV-1 RNA can rebound after suppression in 3 to 6 days after stopping treatment. Adherent patients may experience transient viremia (viral blip) or detectable HIV-1 RNAs in adequately suppressed individuals, that returns to undetectable HIV-1 RNA levels immediately after. These blips are often difficult to diagnose as they can occur between HIV-1 RNA monitoring periods and are identified in a retrospective manner. The 2016 Swedish HIV-cohort retroactively studied the occurrence of blips in 735 subjects between 2007-2013. In these subjects, 10.3% experienced blips with the average blip being 76 copies/mL. This study reported a significant association between the occurrence of viral blip and virologic failure [10]. Though the full clinical significance of viral blips remains uncertain, guidelines recommend providers conduct patient specific adherence assessment after a blip. Patients should be counseled to use secondary methods of sexual prevention for an unspecified period after blip occurrence [3].

In combination with adequate ART-induced HIV-1 RNA suppression, patients should continue use of barrier methods to reduce transmission of sexually transmitted infections (STIs). Though there is no direct association with HIV and STIs, the rate of STIs is growing in the HIV population. The use TasP and PrEP reduce patient concerns about condomless sex with HIV positive partners. Patient attitudes about STI transmission need revisiting, considering these alterations in sexual behaviors [11]. Modified behavior, including condom use, is essential to avoid the acquisition and transmission of STIs. Along with STI prevention, patients should be educated on principles of TasP. These principles are specific to sexual transmission of HIV. The efficacy of this model has not been sufficiently studied in blood exposure transmission. Patients should be counseled that TasP has not been found to reduce transmission during his risk behaviors, such as nonsterile drug injection [3].

The DHHS Guidelines for ARV therapy in adults and adolescents recommend treating most ART-naïve patients with two nucleoside reverse-transcriptase inhibitors (NRTIs) plus an integrase strand transfer Inhibitor (INSTI), a non-nucleoside reverse-transcriptase inhibitor (NNRTI), or a boosted protease inhibitor (PI). INSTI-based regimens have been found to be more tolerable than boosted PI regimens. NNRTI-based regimens are effective, but widespread use has resulted in low barriers to resistance. Recent trials support the initiation of dolutegravir (DTG) plus lamivudine (3TC) in treatment-naïve patients. This regimen was found to be noninferior to a DTG plus tenofovir/emtricitabine (TDF/FTC) regimen. Use of DTG plus 3TC is not appropriate if the patient has HIV-1 RNA >500,000 copies/mL, coinfection with HBV, or HIV genotypic resistance testing or HBV testing has not been made available. Special caution should be used when prescribing DTG and other INSTIs to women of child-bearing age due to recent data from Botswana, reporting an increased risk of neural tube defects in infants born to women who were receiving DTG at the time of conception [12].

Though there are many regimens deemed effective for initial treatment, choice of ART should be made on a risk vs. benefit basis. Assessment of tolerability, toxicity, pill burden and dosing frequency, drug interactions, cost, and evidence-based performance is necessary. DHHS preferred agents for each class are listed in Table 2, and the recommended regimens as initial therapy for most people with HIV are described in Table 3. These combination therapies are preferred due to their durable virologic efficacy in clinical trials, ease of use, and excellent tolerability and toxicity profiles [3].

Table 2. Preferred First Line ARV agents by class [3]

NRTIs	INSTIs	NNRTIs	PIs
abacavir/ lamivudine (ABC/3TC)	bictegravir (BIC)	doravirine (DOR)	atazanavir (ATV)
tenofovir disoproxil fumarate / lamivudine (TDF/3TC)	dolutegravir (DTG)	efavirenz (EFV)	darunavir (DRV)
tenofovir alafenamide/ emtricitabine (TAF/FTC)	elvitegravir/ cobicistat (EVG/c)	rilpivirine (RPV)	
tenofovir disoproxil fumarate/ emtricitabine (TDF/FTC)	raltegravir (RAL)		

Table 3. Recommended ART Combinations as Initial Therapy for Most Persons with HIV [3]

INSTI plus 2 NRTIs
BIC/TAF/FTC
DTG/ABC/3TC – *if HLA-B*5701 negative*
DTG plus (TAF or TDF) plus (FTC or 3TC)
RAL plus (TAF or TDF) plus (FTC or 3TC)
INSTI plus 1 NRTI
DTG/3TC, except for persons with HIV-1 RNA >500,000 copies/mL, HBV coinfection, or if ART must be started before the results of HIV genotypic resistance testing for reverse transcriptase or HBV testing are available

INSTI: integrase strand inhibitor; NRTI: nucleoside reverse transcriptase inhibitor; BIC: bictegravir; TAF: tenofovir alafenamide; FTC: emtricitabine; DTG: dolutegravir; ABC: abacavir; 3TC: lamivudine; TDF: tenofovir disoproxil fumarate; RAL: raltegravir; HBV: hepatitis B virus; ART: antiretroviral therapy.

World Health Organization (WHO)

The WHO recommends HIV prevention efforts be targeted at key populations with increased risk of HIV infection. In 2016 it was estimated the 40 - 50% of worldwide new HIV infections occurred in individuals from key populations. These at-risk communities include MSMs, people who inject drugs, people in prisons and other closed settings, sex workers, and transgender people. Behavioral approaches are key to decreasing the risk of HIV transmission and increase use of recourses in these target groups. The 2016 guidelines list strategies to target these communities including condom promotion programs for sex workers and peer interventions for people who inject illicit drugs [13].

Of the 37.9 million individuals with HIV at the conclusion of 2018, 79% had been diagnosed. In order to increase the number of individuals receiving early ART, the WHO recommends tactics to enhance HIV screening. Countries should develop a standardized HIV screening strategy to provide clear direction to healthcare providers. Accuracy of screening can be improved by moving from a 2 to 3 consecutive reactive test model for diagnosis. Targeting communication through social media is a useful tactic to increase screenings in key populations. Recent Vietnamese studies report that reaching at risk individuals through innovative digital communications led to 95% of those counseled receiving HIV screening. The WHO also recommends integrating screening for other infections to help streamline treatment. Specifically, rapid dual testing of HIV and syphilis should be used first in antenatal period to reduce the rate of infection related stillbirths [14].

HIV self-testing consists of a single rapid diagnostic test of an individual's blood or oral fluid. This method does not offer a definitive HIV-positive diagnosis; however, it can be used to guide at risk persons to seek further screening and treatment if necessary. Patient initiating their own screening will experience increased autonomy through convenience and discretion. Self-testing for HIV has been found to be effective at increasing the frequency of testing and reducing screening-related costs. To advance TasP efforts, guidelines recommend the use of this resource as a gateway to diagnosis for individuals who avoid clinical testing centers [13].

Table 4. World Health Organization First-Line ART Regimens [16]

Population	Preferred 1st line regimen	Alternative 1st line regimen	Special circumstances
Adults and adolescents	TDF+3TC (or FTC)+DTG	TDF+3TC+EFV 400mg	TDF+3TC (or FTC)+EFV 600mg AZT+3TC+EFV 600mg TDF+3TC (or FTC)+PI/r TDF+3TC (or FTC)+RAL TAF+3TC (or FTC)+DTG ABC+3TC+DTG
Children	ABC+3TC+DTG	ABC+3TC+LPV/r ABC+3TC+RAL TAF+3TC (or FTC)+DTG	ABC+3TC+EFV (or NVP) AZT+3TC+EFV (or NVP) AZT+3TC+LPV/r (or RAL)
Neonates	AZT+3TC+RAL	AZT+3TC+NVP	AZT+3TC+LPV/r

3TC: lamivudine; ABC: abacavir; AZT: zidovudine; DTG: dolutegravir; EFV: efavirenz; FTC: emtricitabine; LPV/r: lopinavir/ritonavir; NVP: nevirapine; PI/r: protease inhibitor boosted with ritonavir; RAL: raltegravir; TAF: tenofovir alafenamide; TDF: tenofovir disoproxil fumarate.

The WHO released a 2019 update on the first- and second-line ARV drugs. New guidelines recommend DTG-containing regimens first line due to increasing resistance to NNRTIs. DTG can also be used to treat HIV-2 infection. Children and infants without access to DTG should be treated with a raltegravir-based regimen, first line. After the results of a 2018 observational study in Botswana, DTG therapy became associated with neural tube defects at conception [15]. The 2019 updated publication expressed a lower occurrence of neural tube defects in the Tsepamo study than originally reported, with the rate of 0.30% instead of the 0.94% originally reported in 2018 [12]. The WHO speculates that the rate of neural tube defects in Botswana may have been related to the country's lack of national food folate fortification. DTG initiation can result in greater maternal viral suppression, fewer sexual transmissions and fewer perinatal transmissions.

Use of this agent in women with childbearing potential should be determined by risk to benefits assessment. Recommended first line WHO regimens are described in Table 4 [16].

STRATEGIES TO ENSURE THE SUCCESS OF TASP

The WHO guidelines suggest developing strategies to manage the growth in the population of patients on ART in a TasP model. To ensure quality of care is maintained for all patients, healthcare providers should observe the changes in HIV-1 RNA monitoring. Relaxed monitoring parameters for patients who have achieved consistent HIV-1 RNA suppression will allow providers to allocate time to newly diagnosed and at-risk populations. Adherence to ART is a large factor in the success of the TasP model. In order to achieve an undetectable HIV-1 RNA patient must achieve an adherence level greater than 95%. To promote adherence, it is essential to select ART regimens that have desirable patient-specific tolerability profiles.

Providers should educate patients on expected adverse events of the prescribed ART prior to initiation. Extensive data collection is necessary as ARV tolerability can be influenced by many features including genetic factors and patient lifestyle. Immediately occurring effects can be addressed however, measures to manage ARV effects that occur over long term use should be included in the treatment plan of each patient receiving ART [13, 17].

Treatment guidelines have been updated to usher in the discontinuation of ARV agents that have been to cause interruptions in therapy due to toxicities. Stavudine (d4T) is listed as an agent with recognizable toxicities. After 6 to 12 months of treatment with this thymidine based NRTI patients may experience cumulative mitochondrial toxicity that results in long term lipoatrophy, peripheral neuropathy, lactic acidosis, or pancreatitis. Guidelines offer principles to initiate and achieve the phase out d4T; these include listing azidothymidine (AZT) or TDF based regimens as optimal substitutes for a d4T combination regimen. Patient-specific risk should be evaluated in order to effectively phase out d4T, including evaluation of cost burden associated with discontinuing low cost generic options [16].

With increased life expectancy of HIV infected individuals, the need for low cost ART has been highlighted by guidelines promoting TasP. Adherence to ART depends greatly on the cost and accessibility of the agents.

The global efforts to reduce patient cost burden has resulted in affordable generic ARV drugs in low- and middle-income countries. Providers should be aware of patient economic circumstances when selecting ART. The WHO recommends integration of essential HIV services into national health benefit packages and promoting innovative public/private partnerships to increase availability of ARV. The advancement of these partnerships will depend on funding driven efforts to strengthen laboratory testing networks and the number of qualified providers. Efforts should begin in geographical areas with large amounts of at-risk individuals [13].

TASP CONTROVERSIES

Cost Effectiveness

While cost effectiveness models have found TasP to have high cost burden in the short term, projections into long term use of these principles is expected to be highly cost effective. Methods to evaluate the cost of TasP should include joint measures such as, life-years saved or disability-adjusted life years (DALYs) averted to illustrate the health-related quality of life. Cost analysis of the HPTN 052 and similar trials have estimated favorable cost-effectiveness ratios ranging from $199 per DALY averted to $512 per quality-adjusted life year gained with a TasP model. In Vietnamese studies, the incremental cost per DALY averted was $289 in a population leading in female sex workers, MSM, and injecting drug users. TasP cost burden can be reduced by incorporating task shifting. The tasks of lower level providers should grow in order to allow prioritization in more specialized personnel.

Also, the development of differentiated care will reduce the cost of TasP; this method may include promoting ART adherence monitoring within peer groups, for patients with well suppressed HIV-1 RNAs, to decrease clinical costs [18].

PrEP vs TasP on Rate of New HIV Infections

The use of a tenofovir/emtricitabine (Truvada®) regimen for HIV prevention in at-risk individuals (PrEP) was approved in 2012. In a recent study conducted by Gilead Sciences, it was found that between 2012 and 2017, PrEP contributed 2.1 times that of TasP to the decline in new HIV infections. The effects of PrEP on HIV infections were found to be independent of HIV-1 RNA suppression. These data suggest that the decline in new HIV infections can be attributed to more to PrEP than to TasP efforts. Implications of these results remain to be unseen; however, it should be noted that this study was conducted by the manufacturer of the ARV drugs in PrEP. Also, it may be useful to view these data with the knowledge of PrEP usage rates and the contribution of external factors, such as increased HIV testing, during the 6 years studied [19].

Societal Concerns

Generally, HIV diagnosis and treatment continue to carry a stigma. These negative beliefs and attitudes toward HIV infected individuals can extend to their families and associates. Targeted communities often include gay and bisexual men, homeless people, street youth, the mentally ill, and others who are heavily impacted by HIV. The CDC offers guidance on dealing with the stigma and discrimination associated with increasing HIV treatment.

Patients should be educated on their rights including legislation geared toward promoting the equal rights of those with HIV diagnosis and their associates [20]. Also, increasing public education can reduce misconceptions on the transmission of HIV and the healthcare benefits HIV TasP.

CONCLUSION

TasP is a model that incorporates early diagnosis and immediate ART in order to suppress RNA replication. Maintenance of HIV-1 RNA at less than 200 copies/mL have been found to prevent sexual transmission of HIV from infected individuals. The WHO and DHHS provide guidance on strategies to implement and succeed in HIV prevention with TasP. There may be high cost associated with this method, but the long-term health benefits are great. Studies have shown that the occurrence of new HIV infections declined in recent years. Though this decline cannot be attributed primarily to TasP, it was contributory to these advances in HIV treatment. To ensure success of TasP, healthcare professionals should develop strategies to increase adherence, affordability and availability of ART.

The future of TasP is dependent on the healthcare system's ability to integrate services and set attainable targets. A working example of enacting TasP methods is currently being led by Joint United Nations Programme on HIV/AIDS (UNAIDS). The Fast Track 2020 is a coordinated effort, to end AIDS by 2030. In order to reach this goal providers should aim to achieve 90 – 90 - 90 targets, representing the percentages of HIV positive individuals aware of their status, on ART, and undetectable. It is estimated that reaching these targets will result in less than 500,000 new HIV infections annually by 2020.

UNAIDS projects 95-95 - 95 targets for 2030 that will result in less than 200,000 new HIV infections annually effectively ending the AIDS epidemic [21].

REFERENCES

[1] Centers for Disease Control and Prevention (CDC). *"HIV/AIDS Basics"*. Accessed March 1, 2020. https://www.cdc.gov/hiv/basics/whatishiv.html.

[2] Centers for Disease Control and Prevention (CDC). *"HIV/AIDS Statistics Overview"*. Accessed March 1, 2020. https://www.cdc.gov/hiv/statistics/overview/index.html.

[3] U.S. Department of Health and Human Services (DHHS). *"Guidelines for the Use of Antiretroviral Agents in Adults and Adolescents with HIV"*. Accessed March 1, 2020. https://aidsinfo.nih.gov/guidelines/html/1/adult-and-adolescent-arv/0.

[4] The World Health Organization (WHO). *HIV/AIDS*. Accessed March 1, 2020. https://www.who.int/features/qa/71/en/.

[5] Cohen, M. S., Chen, Y. Q., McCauley, M., Gamble, T., Hosseinipour, M. C., Kumarasamy, N. et al. 2016. "Antiretroviral Therapy for the Prevention of HIV-1 Transmission". *N Engl. J. Med.,* 375: 830 - 9.

[6] Rodger, A. J., Cambiano, V., Bruun, T., Vernazza, P., Collins, S., van Lunzen, J. et al. 2016. "Sexual Activity Without Condoms and Risk of HIV Transmission in Serodifferent Couples When the HIV-Positive Partner Is Using Suppressive Antiretroviral Therapy". *JAMA,* 316: 171 - 81.

[7] Rodger, A. J., Cambiano, V., Bruun, T., Vernazza, P., Collins, S., Degen, O. et al. 2019. "Risk of HIV transmission through condomless sex in serodifferent gay couples with the HIV-positive partner taking suppressive antiretroviral therapy (PARTNER): final

results of a multicentre, prospective, observational study". *Lancet,* 393: 2428 - 38.

[8] Bavinton, B. R., Jin, F., Prestage, G., Zablotska, I., Koelsch, K. K., Phanuphak, N. et al. 2014. "The Opposites Attract Study of viral load, HIV treatment and HIV transmission in serodiscordant homosexual male couples: design and methods". *BMC Public Health,* 14: 917.

[9] Mujugira, A., Celum, C., Coombs, R. W., Campbell, J. D., Ndase, P., Ronald, A. et al. 2016. "HIV Transmission Risk Persists During the First 6 Months of Antiretroviral Therapy". *J. Acquir. Immune Defic. Syndr.,* 72: 579 - 84.

[10] Sorstedt, E., Nilsson, S., Blaxhult, A., Gisslen, M., Flamholc, L. Sonnerborg, A. et al. 2016. "Viral blips during suppressive antiretroviral treatment are associated with high baseline HIV-1 RNA levels". *BMC Infect. Dis.,* 16: 305.

[11] Marrazzo, J. M., Dombrowski, J. C. and Mayer, K. H. 2018. "Sexually transmitted infections in the era of antiretroviral-based HIV prevention: Priorities for discovery research, implementation science, and community involvement". *PLoS Med.,* 15: e1002485.

[12] Zash, R., Holmes, L., Diseko, M., Jacobson, D. L., Brummel, S., Mayondi, G. et al. 2019. "Neural-Tube Defects and Antiretroviral Treatment Regimens in Botswana". *N Engl. J. Med.,* 381: 827 - 40.

[13] The World Health Organization (WHO). *"Consolidated Guidelines on HIV Prevention, Diagnsois, Treatment and Care for Key Populations. 2016 Update".* Accessed March 1, 2020. https://apps.who.int/iris/bitstream/handle/10665/246200/9789241511124-eng.pdf?sequence=8.

[14] The World Health Organization (WHO). *"Innovative WHO HIV Testing Recommendations Aim to Expand Treatment Coverage".* Accessed March 1, 2020. https://www.who.int/news-room/detail/27-11-2019-innovative-who-hiv-testing-recommendations-aim-to-expand-treatment-coverage.

[15] Zash, R., Makhema, J. and Shapiro, R. L. 2018. "Neural-Tube Defects with Dolutegravir Treatment from the Time of Conception". *N Engl. J. Med.*, 379: 979 - 81.

[16] The World Health Organization (WHO). *"Update of Recommendations on First- and Second-Line Antiretroviral Regimens. July 2019"*. Accessed March 1, 2020. https://apps.who.int/iris/bitstream/handle/10665/325892/WHO-CDS-HIV-19.15-eng.pdf?ua=1.

[17] Iacob, S. A., Iacob, D. G. and Jugulete, G. 2017. "Improving the Adherence to Antiretroviral Therapy, a Difficult but Essential Task for a Successful HIV Treatment-Clinical Points of View and Practical Considerations". *Front. Pharmacol.*, 8: 831.

[18] Holmes, C. B., Hallett, T. B., Walensky, R. P., Barnighausen, T., Pillay, Y. and Cohen, M. S. "Effectiveness and Cost-Effectiveness of Treatment as Prevention for HIV". In *Major Infectious Diseases*, edited by rd, K. K. Holmes, S. Bertozzi, B. R. Bloom and P. Jha. Washington (DC), 2017.

[19] Mera-Giler, R., Das, M., Hawkins, T., Asubonteng, J., Magnuson, D., McCallister, S. PrEP Significantly reduces the rate of new HIV diagnoses in US metropolitan statistical areas independent of treatment as prevention (2012 - 2017). Presented at *IDWeek*, October 2 - 6, 2019, Washington, DC. Abstract 1963.

[20] Centers for Disease Control and Prevention (CDC*). "Living with HIV"*. Accessed March 1, 2020. https://www.cdc.gov/hiv/basics/livingwithhiv/stigma-discrimination.html.

[21] Joint United Nations Programme on HIV/AIDS (UNAIDS). *"Understanding Fast-Track. Accelerating Action to End the AIDS Epidemic by 2030"*. Accessed March 1, 2020. https://www.unaids.org/sites/default/files/media_asset/201506_JC2743_Understanding_FastTrack_en.pdf.

INDEX

A

abacavir hypersensitivity reaction,, 102
adherence to treatment, vii, viii, 2, 38
adolescent/youth friendly health services, 124
and counselling, 107, 108, 109
antiretroviral therapy (ART), vii, x, 4, 5, 8, 10, 11, 12, 13, 14, 15, 16, 17, 18, 19, 20, 24, 26, 28, 29, 30, 32, 33, 36, 40, 42, 43, 45, 46, 47, 48, 49, 50, 58, 60, 61, 62, 64, 76, 78, 79, 82, 83, 91, 97, 99, 101, 102, 103, 119, 130, 135, 137, 138, 139, 140, 141, 142, 143, 144, 145, 146, 147, 148, 149, 150, 151, 152, 153, 154
anxiety, v, vii, viii, 1, 3, 4, 5, 6, 7, 8, 9, 12, 14, 15, 16, 17, 18, 19, 20, 21, 22, 23, 24, 25, 26, 27, 28, 29, 30, 31, 33, 36, 37, 38, 39, 40, 42, 43, 44, 45, 46, 47, 48, 49, 50, 51, 52, 53, 54, 57, 62, 65, 66, 67, 116, 123
ARV regimen, 102

B

barriers to ART, 103
behavioural, vii, x, 58, 65, 98, 113, 129
behavioural intervention, 65, 113
benzodiazepines, viii, 2, 30, 38
biomedical, vii, x, 98, 99, 106
biomedical intervention, 99, 106

C

CD4 cells, 99
CD4 T cell count, 99, 100
cell phones, 126, 130
citalopram, viii, 2, 30, 32, 38, 64
client initiated, 107
Clonazepam, viii, 2, 38
Cloud-Native technology, 129
cognitive behavior therapy, viii, 2, 33, 38
cognitive–behavioral stress management, viii, 2, 33, 36, 38
cognitive–behavioral-oriented group psychotherapy, viii, 2, 33, 38
condom effectiveness, 116

Index

cultural reasons, 105

D

dentistry, 70, 77, 78
depression, v, vii, viii, 1, 3, 4, 5, 6, 7, 8, 9, 10, 11, 12, 13, 14, 15, 16, 17, 19, 20, 21, 22, 23, 24, 25, 26, 27, 28, 29, 30, 31, 32, 33, 34, 35, 36, 37, 38, 39, 40, 41, 42, 43, 44, 45, 46, 47, 48, 49, 50, 52, 53, 54, 56, 57, 58, 59, 60, 61, 62, 63, 64, 65, 66, 67, 71, 116, 123
device-based surgical methods, 104
DevOps, 129, 130
discrimination, vii, ix, 14, 33, 52, 57, 69, 70, 71, 72, 73, 74, 75, 76, 77, 79, 109, 119, 120, 121, 122, 124, 134, 151, 154

E

escitalopram, viii, 2, 30, 32, 38
experiential group psychotherapy, viii, 2, 33, 35, 38, 66

F

female condom, 111, 113, 114

G

gender non-conforming, 118, 119

H

high prevalence countries, x, 98
HIV infection, vii, ix, x, 3, 4, 5, 8, 10, 17, 20, 22, 23, 25, 26, 27, 28, 33, 35, 40, 41, 43, 45, 48, 53, 55, 56, 57, 59, 60, 64, 65, 67, 69, 70, 72, 73, 74, 75, 76, 79, 83, 84, 98, 99, 100, 110, 111, 112, 115, 116, 118, 120, 121, 122, 132, 137, 138, 140, 141, 142, 146, 150, 151, 152
HIV related discrimination, 120, 121
HIV status, vii, ix, 8, 51, 70, 71, 73, 74, 75, 103, 106, 107, 108, 110, 120, 121
HIV/AIDS., x, 42, 45, 49, 55, 56, 58, 60, 63, 76, 98, 99, 105, 115, 120, 123, 124, 128, 135, 152
HIV-related stigma, 15, 57, 58, 79, 120
hyper-bilirubinema, 102

I

immune system, 3, 76, 99, 101, 138
indinas (Crixivan), 100
informed consent, 107
innovative technological strategies, x, 98
innovative use of technology, 126
interpersonal therapy, viii, 2, 33, 34, 38

J

judgemental attitudes, 103

L

lorazepam, viii, 2, 30, 38

M

male condom, 113
mindfulness based therapy, 2
morbidity, vii, viii, 2, 4, 12, 38, 42, 44, 55, 56, 60, 72, 99, 103
mortality, 4, 52, 53, 59, 61, 83, 84, 99
multiple partners, 115, 118

O

opportunistic infection, 15, 100, 108, 138

osamprenavir, 100
overcoming, 76, 110

P

people living with HIV/AIDS, vii, viii, ix, 2, 4, 38, 39, 40, 42, 43, 44, 45, 47, 48, 49, 51, 52, 57, 67, 70, 73, 75, 77, 78, 79, 94
physical barrier, 111, 113
post-test counselling, 109
pre-existing biases, 120
Previstaf, 100
prophylactic drugs, 108
protease inhibitors, 30, 86, 92, 102
provider initiated testing, 107

R

religious, 104, 105, 112, 116, 117, 119, 123
risky sexual behaviours, 113, 117, 120, 122
rite of passage to adulthood, 105

S

selective serotonin reuptake inhibitors, 2, 31
self-destructive behaviours, x, 98
sertraline, viii, 2, 30, 32, 38
sexual behavioural change, 110
sexual debut, 115, 117, 118, 134
sexual dysfunction, 5, 9, 17, 20, 31, 33
sexuality and sexual identity, 117
sexually active, x, 98, 115, 118
sexually transmitted infections, x, 98, 105, 143
sexually vulnerable, 118
social media, 125, 126, 127, 135, 146
social stigma, 5, 132
societal level factors, 121

stigma, vii, viii, 9, 11, 12, 15, 16, 18, 20, 22, 26, 33, 45, 57, 69, 70, 71, 73, 74, 75, 76, 77, 78, 79, 103, 109, 116, 119, 120, 121, 122, 123, 124, 131, 132, 133, 134, 150, 154
stress management, viii, 2, 33, 36, 38, 66, 67
structural intervention, x, 98, 120
structural interventions, x, 98
sub-Saharan Africa (SSA), x, 44, 51, 97, 98, 101, 106
supportive psychotherapy, viii, 2, 33, 34, 35, 38

T

toxicities, 102, 148
tricyclic antidepressants, 2, 32, 64

U

United Nations Programme on HIV/AIDS (UNAIDS), x, 70, 71, 75, 79, 98, 99, 104, 106, 107, 135, 151, 152, 154

V

vaginal microbicides, 99, 110, 111
voluntary male circumcision, 99, 103
vulnerable groups, 110

W

woman-initiated prevention strategy, 110
World Health Organization (WHO), x, 3, 6, 15, 22, 39, 70, 72, 80, 82, 93, 98, 102, 103, 104, 111, 124, 132, 136, 137, 146, 147, 148, 149, 151, 152, 153, 154